# Contents

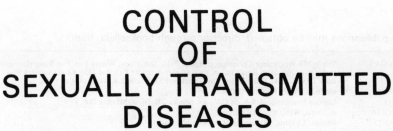

# CONTROL
# OF
# SEXUALLY TRANSMITTED
# DISEASES

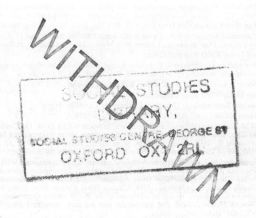

## GENEVA
## WORLD HEALTH ORGANIZATION
## 1985

ISBN 92 4 154198 9

World Health Organization 1985

TYPESET IN INDIA
PRINTED IN ENGLAND

83/5900-Macmillan/Spottiswoode-7000

# Preface

The prevalence of sexually transmitted diseases has reached a disturbing level in many countries and the World Health Organization has alerted its Members to the gravity of the complications that may arise if these diseases are not treated adequately and at an early stage. These complications can have serious consequences for the individual, the family, and the community.

The present situation has arisen not as a result of a lack of knowledge or a shortage of resources but because in many countries there has been (1) inadequate use of well-established techniques, (2) poor monitoring and poor evaluation of control, and (3) an incorrect social and educational approach. In order to achieve the goal of health for all by the year 2000 set by WHO's Member States, this public health problem must be tackled by a multidisciplinary approach involving coordinated action by health personnel at all levels, and by the health education, information, and welfare services.

In response to the current situation, and to requests from the World Health Assembly, three WHO Scientific Groups have examined different technical aspects of the problem and their reports have been published in the *Technical Report Series*. The present book has been prepared following the meeting of a scientific working group that was held in Washington in April 1982 to discuss the formulation of appropriate strategies and programmes for the control of this group of diseases.[1] This book emphasizes the need for such programmes to be integrated into general programmes for the control of communicable diseases and for the gynaecological, obstetric, paediatric, and urological services to play an active and dynamic part.

---

[1] A list of the participants in the scientific working group is given in Annex 6, page 109.

# Chapter 1. Introduction

The greater attention being given to the control of sexually transmitted diseases in many countries reflects the increasing prevalence of these diseases, their adverse health effects, and the greater capability of the countries to address these problems. The technical aspects of the main sexually transmitted diseases have been considered in the reports of three WHO Scientific Groups (1–3) and the present book is concerned with control strategies and programmes.

## 1.1 Terminology

A control activity for sexually transmitted diseases is any activity which minimizes the adverse health effects of this group of diseases. Control activities may reduce (a) the incidence of disease; (b) the duration of the disease; (c) the effects of each case, including both the physical complications and psychosocial consequences; or (d) the cost of achieving certain outcomes, i.e., increase the efficiency of services. Many different control activities, for example, clinical services, screening, and contact tracing, can reduce the effects of sexually transmitted diseases.

A control programme is composed of various control activities. Priorities are established, various options for control are examined, and appropriate methods are adopted. Such a programme will achieve its objectives by the design and implementation of work plans. Evaluation is used to reveal any need for programme change. These alterations may be needed because the programme is ineffective or because changes have occurred in the diseases, their setting, or the opportunities for intervention.

The epidemiology of sexually transmitted diseases and their associated complications is very variable. In addition, for each facet of the problem, the effectiveness of particular control activities is different. At the planning stage, the expected health effects of control activities should be specified as clearly as possible. Such planning will clarify the control decisions made and justify the programme activities. Furthermore, specification of the activities in the initial stages will facilitate the integration of the control programme into the overall health scheme. Clearly written plans will identify the many components of the control programme within the health system, thus facilitating the evaluation process.

Control programmes for sexually transmitted diseases define the population to be covered and specify the control activities related to that group. For instance, some programmes to control congenital syphilis specify that all pregnant women are to be included, to ensure that they undergo antenatal examination and are serologically tested and treated if necessary. However, coverage of the target population may be incomplete

1

and performance of the specified activities inaccurate. Some pregnant women will not attend antenatal facilities or will attend either late in their pregnancy or only sporadically; serological tests will be omitted on occasions; and some serological reactors will deliver their babies without having had treatment. However, when the target population and the particular activities to be undertaken are clearly defined, the step(s) at which serious performance problems occur can be readily identified. Once identified, the reasons for the performance problems can be sought and programme changes can then be made.

In contrast, services for sexually transmitted diseases are those made available to self-selected individuals from the overall population. The diseases seen by such services may, however, differ from those of the overall population, and the differences are likely to be greater when services are less readily available. Although services and programmes are distinct, services of some type will always be part of a control programme. Therefore, control programmes for sexually transmitted diseases must encourage continued improvements in these services and seek ways to enhance their contribution to the control effort.

## 1.2 Approaches to control

Effective efforts to control sexually transmitted diseases must be appropriate to the unique settings, populations, and disease problems of each programme. Thus, the design and format of each control programme will be unique and cannot be transferred from one setting to another without careful adaptation. Extremes in control programmes can be grouped as follows: (a) categorical or vertical control programmes; and (b) integrated or horizontal control programmes. In practice, however, effective categorical programmes are also integrated into the general health and social systems of a country and depend upon them for their functioning. In order to develop and adapt efficiently with time, effective integrated programmes depend upon the availability of suitable expertise, either local or foreign. The choice is not, therefore, one of categorical versus integrated control programmes for sexually transmitted diseases, but rather is one of determining the mixture of categorical expertise and general health system integration within each setting.

## 1.3 Control programme planning

At the simplest level, control programme planning is designed to ensure that the highest priority disease or problem is identified and that resources are not wasted on activities that are too costly or are inappropriate. The general questions that must be answered are: (a) which disease or problem is the most serious and important to the government, the public, and the health system; (b) can the health effects of the identified problem(s) be reduced by low-cost activities; (c) what would be the result of such activities; (*d*) what resources would be needed to implement them and are they available; and (*e*) how could the effects of these activities be measured? The answers to these questions will define the focus of a new programme or a new element for an existing programme and will determine whether a given activity should be attempted. Before implementation, the programme manager should develop a timetable for the review of the activity. This review should specify unambiguous guidelines for the continuance, modification, or cessation of the activity depending on the findings.

*Formal control plans*

More formal programme planning is appropriate when categorical control staff exist and skilled epidemiological and management resources are available. Such planning may include the following seven elements.

(1) *Problem definition*. Clarification of the problems posed by sexually transmitted diseases includes a description of the occurrence of disease, disease prevalence and any possible complications by area and population groups. The adverse health effects of these diseases will generally be increased for specific groups and geographical areas and thus the identification of these provides a focus for the control efforts. Similarly, disease transmission is not the same throughout the infected population; information that identifies the important transmitter groups may be needed in order to interrupt disease transmission more efficiently.

Information in these areas is inadequate or non-existent in most cases. Initial programme considerations must clarify what data are available and improve the data collection, analysis, and use. The construction of a model of the transmission of disease and the development of complications, and their control, may be helpful in considering the disease problem and programme activities (*4*). Different models can be developed to consider other problems such as congenital syphilis, in which the issues are related to pregnancy, and hepatitis B in which intervention with a vaccine can be considered.

(2) *Establishing priorities*. The priorities for control begin with the health problem description. The availability of adequate resources must be identified for various possible interventions. The commitment of the government and of the health staff in particular, will also be crucial in the selection of priority problems and interventions. Finally, public commitment to the control effort must be assessed in order to identify the nature and degree of support that might be expected. Thus, the control priorities selected will be an amalgam of health problem considerations and control feasibility.

(3) *Setting objectives*. Objectives are a statement of the intention of the control programme to reduce the health effects of sexually transmitted diseases within a given population and a stated time. Programme success can be defined as the degree to which its objectives are met. To be most useful, objectives should be unambiguous and quantifiable.

Programme objectives that are simple and realistic, i.e., that can be achieved within the proposed time and setting, are more helpful than those which are grandiose or broad. For instance, an objective "to reduce the prevalence and incidence of disease" is not helpful in designing or evaluating control efforts unless more details of this general, long-range objective are specified and can be measured.

(4) *Considering strategies.* A variety of intervention strategies for the control of sexually transmitted diseases exists. Each strategy has different resource requirements and effects; these should be reviewed in light of the programme objectives, target population(s), and proposed timetable. Ideally, planners should perform a cost-benefit or a cost-effectiveness analysis of alternative strategies to select the most effective, feasible strategy. In practical terms, an estimate of desirable outcomes (effectiveness) and of possible costs is often all that is available to make initial programme decisions. Control programmes generally use more than one strategy; planners must determine the mixture of strategies that appears to be most appropriate to the setting.

(5) *Planning for implementation.* A written plan, reflecting the problem, the objectives, and the strategies, which also details the activities required and the timetable for implementation, is useful to the programme manager. Development of such a plan will encourage careful consideration of the resource requirements (both personnel and material), personnel development, and the sequence of development both by area and activity. Such a plan will provide the basis for developing or modifying job descriptions for programme personnel and others who will assist in implementation.

(6) *Planning for evaluation.* Evaluation of a control programme is an integral part of the overall implementation plan, but because of its importance it is often considered separately. Evaluation is used to answer the questions: have the objectives been achieved (outcome) and have the activities been performed as specified (process)? Evaluation should be performed at points that will identify promptly any barriers to implementation. The findings may lead to modification of the programme, extension to new areas or new problems, or the cessation of activities.

(7) *Ensuring operational research.* Barriers encountered in defining the problem, selecting strategies, or meeting evaluation goals will identify areas for operational research. Since such research activities are predicated on solving important programme problems, they should be planned to provide timely feedback to the control programme. As the problems or settings (including technological developments) change, other research topics may assume high priority.

*Programme check-list*

Control programmes for sexually transmitted diseases will be guided by the following considerations: (*a*) adequate provision must be made for planning, implementing, and evaluating the programme, and information needs must be clearly defined at each step; (*b*) programme objectives must be clearly stated and quantified where appropriate and possible; (*c*) alternative strategies must be considered; inappropriate ones must be dropped, some may be deferred pending review of results of initial efforts, and those most likely to be effective must be chosen for implementation; (d) the plan for implementation must be realistic and include a timetable; and (e) appropriate criteria must be chosen for programme evaluation.

## 1.4 Conclusions

In this book various aspects of the control process are considered and it is intended to assist managers in developing or modifying control programmes in many settings. Control programme settings are characterized by very different social and health systems. Thus, there is no inherently correct programme for all settings, even where the disease problems are similar. Furthermore, a control programme for sexually transmitted diseases that is appropriate for a society at one time is unlikely to be appropriate for ever. Societies, health care systems, disease problems, and intervention opportunities are constantly changing. Control programmes must evolve to meet these new challenges and to use the opportunities provided by new interventions. Despite the many differences that exist between countries, all share a lack of public awareness of the magnitude of the problem posed by sexually transmitted diseases.

This book may appear to suggest that the disease control process should be highly systematic, comprehensive, and compartmentalized. In practice, however, many activities take place simultaneously and in a manner that is far from systematic, sequential, and ordered. In addition, the control components and support activities are presented as discrete items. No relative weighting of these efforts is intended; in fact, each effort may be less effective on its own than when it is combined with one or more others.

The control process has been described with some degree of abstraction, avoiding areas of ignorance in order to provide perspective and a sound theoretical framework. It is hoped that this will assist managers to produce a programme that is comprehensive and carefully adapted to the setting.

This book will have an impact on control efforts only when the principles and guidelines described are incorporated into individual programmes. To facilitate this goal the broadest possible support must be sought, ranging from those with responsibility in an individual health programme to those with international or multinational responsibilities. Some actions that will promote control efforts include:

(1) National initiatives that include a wide range of groups and individuals involved in the control of sexually transmitted diseases and that result in the development of appropriate guidelines for that particular country. Where appropriate, these efforts should demonstrate the effectiveness of community participation in control efforts. The expressed needs of the community can be emphasized and reflected in the development of local resources to assist in meeting these needs.

(2) International initiatives on a regional basis should focus on management workshops for the countries of that region. Such programmes

should concentrate on planning, management, and evaluation and encourage the sharing of experiences from the participating countries in each area.

(3) Regional activities should also include a limited number of national pilot control programme projects in different social and health care systems. Such projects may be a prerequisite for significant progress in disease control. These should be designed to demonstrate further that well-planned and carefully evaluated programmes are feasible. Such pilot projects can serve as control models for neighbouring countries. These will be more complete and more readily assimilated than written guidelines. Finally, such pilot projects can help to consolidate and expand the control efforts in the countries in which they are initiated. Obviously such projects will need international, regional, and national support.

(4) Prototype documents for the operation of certain control activities need to be made widely available so that they can be used as guidelines by other programmes. Some such documents are already available (5). Additional prototypes must be developed, tested, and disseminated. These may be developed by consultant groups or may be a major focus of the pilot projects.

## References

1. Technical Report Series No. 616, 1978 (Neisseria gonorrhoeae *and gonococcal infections*: report of a WHO Scientific Group).
2. Technical Report Series No. 660, 1981 (*Nongonococcal urethritis and other selected sexually transmitted diseases of public health importance*: report of a WHO Scientific Group).
3. Technical Report Series No. 674, 1982 (*Treponemal infections*: report of a WHO Scientific Group).
4. HART, G. *Sexual maladjustment and disease. An introduction to modern venereology.* Chicago, Nelson-Hall, 1977, Fig. 12–5, p. 184.
5. CENTERS FOR DISEASE CONTROL. Sexually transmitted diseases. Treatment guidelines 1982. *Morbidity and mortality weekly report*, Vol. 31, No. 25 (1982).

# PART I

# INITIAL PLANNING STEPS

The first step in planning a new control programme for sexually transmitted diseases or in revising an existing programme is to estimate the disease problem by describing the incidence and/or prevalence of each disease and its complications (Chapter 2). Such a description may use available information and/or new information obtained from special studies. Groups at particular risk of having, acquiring, or transmitting a disease and/or suffering the complications of a disease, should also be identified (Chapter 3). Identification of such priority groups will facilitate the selection of strategies and the development of the intervention plans. Finally, geographical or political areas with a particularly severe problem of sexually transmitted diseases should be identified to facilitate the directing of early intervention activities.

The next step in the programme planning process is an attempt to set control priorities. Although control priorities begin with a description of the disease problem, they must also reflect government and public commitment, resources, and technical feasibility. Government commitment to this control activity must be established, including an assessment of the personnel, resources, and supportive activities available from the government. The degree of commitment by the public to control efforts must also be identified and the particular focus of the public's interest must be carefully considered. In order to clarify important aspects of control programmes, sociological aspects of control may be reviewed (Chapter 4). Finally, the technical feasibility of control must be evaluated in order to establish priorities. Unless the necessary technical capability exists or can be established in the country, a particular problem cannot be accorded a high control priority. All these factors—health problems, government and public commitment, and technical feasibility—must be considered together. A study of both the health problems and control feasibility will thus be necessary in order to define the control priorities of the programme.

The final step of the initial planning effort is a statement of the programme objectives to reduce the adverse health effects of sexually transmitted diseases. These objectives will help to identify the target population and the period over which an improvement in their health status is expected to take place.

# Chapter 2. Estimating the public health importance of sexually transmitted diseases

## 2.1 Introduction

Until sexually transmitted diseases are recognized as an important public health problem, only limited resources will be allocated for their control or study. When resources are scarce their epidemiology cannot be studied fully—consequently programme managers encounter difficulties in describing the importance of sexually transmitted diseases and have problems in efficiently using the scarce resources that are available. It is crucial that the public health importance of these diseases is estimated in order to break this vicious cycle of under-funding, inadequate knowledge, limited appreciation of control importance, and hence continued under-funding (1). Preliminary estimates of the importance of these diseases will be used in initial planning steps; more definite descriptions of disease epidemiology will be developed as is necessary for the further development of the programme.

One of the first steps of control planning is to establish why a given sexually transmitted disease is important in a particular country. This process will help to focus the efforts of the control programme staff during preliminary planning and will reveal to decision-makers the priority issues of control. For example, in some countries, gonorrhoea is important because it causes pelvic inflammatory disease (PID) (2). Elsewhere, gonorrhoea is important because the disease is resistant to the available inexpensive antimicrobial drugs (3). Syphilis is important in some countries because it is a common cause of pregnancy wastage (4, 5). However, in other countries, the late manifestations of syphilis have received the most emphasis in programme justification (6).

The preliminary estimates of the importance of a particular disease will also be used to convince decision-makers of the need to allocate new resources to the control programme. Such resources will be essential in developing a clearer, quantitative description of the specific problem and its distribution. These further details of disease epidemiology are required to design an efficient control programme.

## 2.2 Approaches to estimating public health importance

Various approaches may be used to estimate the importance of sexually transmitted diseases and the choice depends on the ingenuity of the manager, the resources available, and the particular disease problems. In addition, the selection of a particular approach to demonstrate the disease's importance depends upon which method will most effectively influence the key decision-makers. These approaches are usually combined in presentations; different aspects of the problem are emphasized depending on the composition of the intended audience.

*Economic consequences*

The economic consequences of sexually transmitted diseases may be used to persuade fiscally-oriented decision-makers that these problems are of considerable importance to public health. The cost of these diseases results in part from direct costs, i.e., the cost of care for patients with either uncomplicated or complicated disease. The major economic burden of these diseases results from the costs involved in caring for patients with disease complications; consequently, the economic costs of disease without complications are much lower. The indirect costs include productivity losses resulting from sick leave, disabilities, or premature death. Again these indirect costs are principally due to disease complications.

In the United States of America (2), using a combination of estimates —data from limited studies (7) and data from national samples—it was calculated that the costs of pelvic inflammatory disease that could be attributed to sexually transmitted diseases amounted to nearly US$ 1.2 billion in 1979. Insufficient data is available in most countries on which to base such a calculation.

*Social consequences*

In countries where sexually transmitted diseases are accompanied by socially important consequences, emphasis on these particular issues will be relevant. The importance of these diseases in causing infertility, fetal wastage, neonatal death and disabilities in children should be emphasized. Data linking particular diseases to these outcomes may need to be strengthened and more widely publicized. In addition, the chronic pain, disability, and pelvic inflammatory disease-related deaths which affect women and interfere with their contribution to a healthy family unit should be highlighted. It may be necessary to emphasize the social consequences of sexually transmitted diseases in order to facilitate discussion of their control by the public and politicians.

*Prediction of future importance*

Demographic, sociological, and behavioural changes occurring throughout the world contribute to the growing importance of these diseases and will continue to do so in the near future. The number of young adults in the population is increasing in most countries, and populations are shifting from rural, traditional areas to urban settings. Family and community ties are changing; consequently there is diminished social control over the behaviour of young adults and they are becoming increasingly sexually active. Thus, more people are at risk of contracting a sexually transmitted disease than ever before and these trends seem likely to continue.

The importance of these diseases relative to other public health problems is also likely to increase. Thus, increasing recognition of the common, serious sequelae of sexually transmitted diseases, e.g., pelvic inflammatory disease, infertility, and pregnancy wastage, will increase the relative importance of these problems. Similarly, increases in the resistance of gonococci to antibiotics and decreases in gonorrhoea therapy response rates emphasize the importance of dealing with these problems before they worsen. The methods of control are rapidly changing, and as the non-cultural diagnostic methods currently under investigation become available, as new vaccines are developed, and as novel therapeutic agents are produced, many possibilities of disease control will become more feasible.

*Opportunities*

Missed opportunities plague public health practitioners. The opportunities to prevent sexually transmitted diseases and their complications should be stressed as an integral part of the effort to ensure that each country achieves the goal of health for all by the year 2000. Efforts to expand the quality and coverage of antenatal and delivery care programmes can be enhanced with improved syphilis screening efforts and innovative approaches to prevent disease-related postpartum sepsis. Family planning programmes should be used to prevent the disease complications of intrauterine contraceptive devices and to detect and treat lower genital tract infections before pelvic inflammatory disease occurs. Where symptomatic genital tract disease is found to be a problem, primary health care workers can be trained to deal with sexually transmitted diseases. The effectiveness of this approach can be improved if the training includes the provision of information concerning the consequences of sexually transmitted diseases and the methods to avoid contracting them. Further, they can encourage the treatment of sexual partners which will limit disease transmission and complications. Since this group of diseases principally affects young people who will be the leaders and parents of the next generation, such preventive measures may be particularly valuable for the future wellbeing of the community.

## 2.3 Guidelines for estimating the importance of sexually transmitted diseases

The preparation of a preliminary estimate of the disease problem is both a political and technical exercise. As a political statement, this estimate will emphasize the particular problems that are most relevant to an important group of decision-makers, and will highlight important issues for the public. As a technical exercise, it will assist in selecting the priorities for subsequent efforts.

Often the necessary data will not be available or, if available, the focus of the problem will be unclear. In such situations, it may be useful to assemble a multidisciplinary group to assist in estimating the problem. Such a group will have access to a variety of data and opinions. The group members should include people from the government health care system, the academic medical community, non-governmental care systems, and others, e.g., sociologists, teachers, statisticians. This group should review available information and develop a consensus opinion, perhaps employing a formalized Delphi method (8). Whether the method depends largely on the analysis of data or upon consensus development based on opinions, this information must be disseminated to have an impact on existing

## Table 1. Special studies to estimate the importance of syphilis

*Fetal wastage*
– Descriptive epidemiology and etiology of abortions, stillbirths, and early neonatal death
– Case-control studies of abortions, stillbirths, and early neonatal deaths
– Descriptive epidemiology of syphilis in pregnancy

*Infertility*
– Case-control studies of infertility

*Genital ulcer disease*
– Descriptive epidemiology and etiology of genital ulcer disease
– Case-control studies of genital ulcer disease

*Late sequelae of syphilis*
– Descriptive epidemiology and etiology of selected diseases
– Case-control studies of indicator diseases
– Descriptive studies of the costs of care associated with indicator diseases

## Table 2. Special studies to estimate the importance of gonorrhoea

*Urethritis and vaginitis*
– Descriptive epidemiology and etiology of urethritis and vaginitis
– Case-control studies of urethritis and vaginitis

*Pelvic inflammatory disease (PID)*
– Descriptive epidemiology and etiology and acute PID
– Case-control studies of acute PID
– Descriptive studies of cases of acute PID
– Descriptive studies of the costs of care associated with PID

*Ophthalmia neonatorum*
– Descriptive epidemiology and etiology of ophthalmia neonatorum
– Case-control studies of ophthalmia neonatorum

*Infertility*
– Descriptive epidemiology of infertility
– Case-control studies of infertility
– Case-control studies of ectopic pregnancies
– Case-control studies of urethral strictures

*Gonococcal resistance*
– Descriptive epidemiology of gonococcal resistance
– Trends of gonococcal resistance

perceptions. The multidisciplinary nature of the group could be useful for facilitating this dissemination to a variety of decision-making groups, both those of the general public and key individuals.

A variety of special studies may be necessary to provide the information needed to make useful statements of importance, in particular for gonorrhoea and syphilis (Tables 1 and 2). The time and resources needed for such studies should be considered before deciding whether they are essential for the formulation of preliminary estimates of the importance of particular sexually transmitted diseases.

## References

1. WILLCOX, R. R. VD education in developing countries. A comparison with developed countries. *British journal of venereal diseases*, **52**: 88–93 (1976).
2. CURRAN, J. W. Economic consequences of pelvic inflammatory disease in the United States. *American journal of obstetrics and gynecology*, **138**: 848–851 (1980).
3. PANIKABUTRA, K. ET AL. Sensitivity to penicillin, thiamphenicol, kanamycin, cefoxitin and spectinomycin of penicillinase-producing *Neisseria gonorrhoeae* (PPNG) in Bangkok. Relation to the results of treatment. *Journal of the Medical Association of Thailand*, **65**: 316–324 (1982).
4. RATNAM, A. V. ET AL. Syphilis in pregnant women in Zambia. *British journal of venereal diseases*, **58**: 355–358 (1982).
5. NAEYE, R. L. ET AL. Causes of perinatal mortality in an African city. *Bulletin of the World Health Organization*, **55**: 63–65 (1977).
6. PARRAN, T. *Shadow in the land: syphilis*. New York, Reynal and Hitchcock, 1937.
7. RENDTORFF, R. C. ET AL. Economic consequences of gonorrhea in women: Experience from an urban hospital. *Journal of American Venereal Disease Association*. **1**: 40–47 (1974).
8. KOPLAN, J. P. & FARER, L. S. Choice of preventive treatment for isoniazid-resistant tuberculosis infection. Use of decision analysis and Delphi technique. *Journal of the American Medical Association*, **244**: 2736–2740 (1980).

# Chapter 3. Priority groups

## 3.1 Introduction

An underlying principle of disease epidemiology is that disease and disease complications are not evenly distributed throughout populations. As a result, some population groups are of greater importance to prevention and control efforts than others. Programme managers must identify such priority groups in order to make efficient use of the scarce control resources. In addition, detailed descriptions of these priority groups may suggest the dynamics of disease within the community and can lead to the development of new intervention activities.

Generally, these priority groups are characterized on the basis of prevalence studies indicating that the proportion of infected individuals in one group is greater than the general population or reference group. More recent emphasis on the "core group" of disease transmitters suggests that a subgroup of infected persons is responsible for the perpetuation of a disease within a community (1, 2). Thus, not all infected individuals are of equal importance to the control programme. Since major emphasis is given in many control programmes to the complications of sexually transmitted diseases, it is logical to focus on another subgroup of individuals i.e., those who suffer complications. Thus, in both developed and developing countries, young women of certain sociocultural subgroups are at greater than average risk of contracting pelvic inflammatory disease (3, 4).

The approach used to categorize population subgroups and to infer causal relationships will be based on the resources available for data collection and analysis.

## 3.2 Priority group descriptions

Priority groups may be categorized on the basis of age, sex, and ethnic group. However, priority groups categorized by these characteristics are generally too broad to be of any great use to control programme managers. Descriptions that also include place of residence or an occupation may be much more helpful in designing interventions (5), and such information is relatively simple to collect and not, in general, stigmatizing. In addition, control activities can be aimed at one particular area of a city or at specific work groups, e.g., the military or students, if such characteristics identify priority groups.

Other characteristics that may be used to identify priority groups include their general health promotion and their sexual and health care-seeking behaviour. This information is more difficult to collect since it is not used as often and is less well standardized. In addition, some responses

14

are stigmatizing, e.g., use of tobacco, alcohol, and drugs, and sexual behaviour. Despite these drawbacks, such definitions of priority groups may be most valuable. Some control programmes have been able to use such behavioural characteristics to identify priority groups. Using this information effectively, very specific intervention activities have been developed in different settings for prostitutes (6, 7) and for homosexuals (8).

## 3.3 Use of defined priority groups

When priority groups are defined, the problems of each group with respect to sexually transmitted diseases can be described more precisely and compared with those of other groups. Such a comparison of groups may lead to further refinement of the priority group definition and may identify disease problems that are peculiar to those groups. This further description of priority groups may also offer insight into those groups and their patterns of behaviour and interactions that may be useful in designing specific control efforts.

Interventions developed for specific priority groups and settings will be unique. The appropriate mix of control elements will depend upon the judgement of health workers who are thoroughly familiar with the available strategies, resources, and the priority groups. Once targeted control activities are outlined, it will be vital to identify and work closely with those individuals who can facilitate interactions with the priority groups. Cooperative ventures developed with priority groups may be a particularly useful approach to ensure collaboration.

## 3.4 Conclusions

A general set of guidelines is proposed for priority groups. The priority groups must be defined, either on the basis of observational anecdotes or by analysis of data. Small-scale surveys or more detailed data collection and analysis will be appropriate in different countries. Specific intervention activities for these groups can then be developed, implemented, and evaluated.

Programme managers must ensure that the process of defining priority groups does not further stigmatize the group. Activities implemented for the priority groups must also be carefully monitored to ensure that these efforts do not defeat the goals of the programme either by alienating priority groups or by suggesting that the disease is a problem caused by the priority group.

## References

1. YORKE, J. A. ET AL. Dynamics and control of the transmission of gonorrhoea. *Sexually transmitted diseases*, **5**: 51–56 (1978).
2. PHILLIPS, L. ET AL. Focussed interviewing in gonorrhoea control. *American journal of public health*, **70**: 705–708 (1980).

3. MUIR, D. G. & BELSEY, M. A. Pelvic inflammatory disease and its consequences in the developing world. *American journal of obstetrics and gynecology*, **183**: 913–928 (1980).
4. ST. JOHN, R. K. ET AL. Pelvic inflammatory disease in the United States: Epidemiology and trends among hospitalized women. *Sexually transmitted diseases*, **8**: 62–66 (1981).
5. ROTHENBERG, R. R. *Analysis of gonorrhea morbidity data.* Paper presented at First World STD Conference. San Juan, Puerto Rico, November 15, 1981.
6. JAFFE, H. W. ET AL. Selective mass treatment in a venereal disease control program. *American journal of public health*, **69**: 181–182 (1979).
7. RAJAN, V. S. Problems in the surveillance and control of sexually transmitted agents associated with pelvic inflammatory disease in the Far East. *American journal of obstetrics and gynecology*, **138**: 1071–1077 (1980).
8. OSTROW, D. G. Homosexuality and STD. In: Holmes, K. K. et al., ed. *Sexually transmitted diseases.* New York, McGraw-Hill, 1984.

# Chapter 4. Sociological aspects of control

## 4.1 Introduction

The problem of the prevention and control of sexually transmitted diseases can be thought of as a social problem with very important medical aspects. Social problems involve personal interactions. Perhaps the most important relationships include: (*a*) clinicians interacting with patients and control personnel; (*b*) priority group members interacting with other persons, clinicians, and control personnel; (*c*) infected persons interacting with clinicians, control personnel, and sexual partners.

This chapter reviews the cultural, social structure, and psychological factors that influence these interactions. Although control programmes cannot attempt to delineate the relevant details of all these factors, consideration of them can enhance the planning process or provide insight into programme performance problems.

## 4.2. Cultural factors

Culture can be described as the accumulated knowledge, beliefs, and values of a social system. Disease prevention and control programmes should be designed, implemented, and evaluated within a given social setting by persons from that social setting. Programme managers will have an innate understanding of their own culture but will inevitably understand some parts of that culture more thoroughly than others. However, this understanding often fails to distinguish between knowledge, beliefs, and values. Such distinctions may prove useful when reviewing why interaction problems exist within the programme.

### Knowledge

Some cultures acknowledge that sexually transmitted diseases are a serious health problem, that these diseases are spread by sexual intercourse, and that they can be controlled through coordinated, purposeful interactions. However, most cultures fail to acknowledge the truth of one or more of these statements. Many studies have shown that education is an effective method of providing information about sexually transmitted diseases (*1, 2*). Such education efforts should be developed around socially acceptable, reasonable, and meaningful objectives (*3*).

17

*Beliefs*

People have faith in beliefs, whether they are true or not. Some believe that sexually transmitted diseases are restricted to promiscuous individuals and fail to realize that innocent spouses and children can become infected. Others pessimistically believe that political leaders cannot be encouraged to support programmes that carry the stigma of these diseases when experiences in Singapore and the United States of America suggest otherwise. Beliefs about personal disease susceptibility, the value of a particular preventive act, and the general importance of staying healthy are probably the critical determinants of behavioural patterns. Individuals' knowledge about germs, the value of prophylactic devices, and the dangers of asymptomatic infections are probably much less important in determining behaviour (4).

The health-belief model was developed to explain why some people accepted recommended health behaviour and others did not (5). Thus, as the model predicted, people who believed that they were susceptible to infections, that sexually transmitted diseases were serious, and that condoms could prevent disease transmission were more likely to have used condoms (6). However, in prospective studies, these same beliefs were not related to future condom use. Although the individuals' beliefs favoured condom use, factors in addition to both belief and knowledge also influenced behaviour.

*Values*

Values refer to things people consider to be relatively desirable, and these values are used to help people choose between alternative courses of action (7). For example, some people choose sexual relationships where there is a risk of contracting disease rather than abstaining or choosing sex without any risk. Some policy-makers support child and maternal health care programmes but do not value the control programmes for sexually transmitted diseases which can prevent the sequelae of pelvic inflammatory disease, pregnancy wastage, neonatal deaths, and congenital disabilities.

Health is valued more by those who do not enjoy it than by those who are healthy. Consequently, few healthy adolescents fear the possibility of disease when they begin experimenting in sexual activities with their peers. Conversely, diseased individuals may, for a period of time, avoid contracting further disease. Thus, patients may be the most important group to educate because some will become advocates of healthy behaviour.

## 4.3 Social-structural factors

Most societies are organized and structured in such a way that some individuals have greater opportunities to achieve their goals than others. These individuals, the community and political leaders, are often responsible for allocating scarce resources. These leaders must be identified and induced to adopt or adapt programme goals as their own so that prevention and control programmes can obtain the necessary resources. Where these leaders have been previously opposed to programme goals, it may be more rewarding to approach somewhat less powerful individuals who have been generally supportive of allied programmes in the past.

Priority groups within societies will place themselves at greater risk of contracting, harbouring, transmitting, or suffering from venereal infection than others for a variety of reasons (Chapter 3). Sociodemographic variables can be extremely helpful in identifying those groups, while a study of their social interactions and social structures may be important in describing these reasons. Such an understanding may be necessary to improve interventions with these groups. In order to minimize disease transmission, reinfections, and complications, public health workers may need to study both the technical aspects of the diseases and the social-structural setting of priority groups.

## 4.4 Psychological factors

Cultural and social factors provide a setting for individuals. However, behavioural decisions may also be made that are other than those predicted on the basis of these factors. Psychological factors relating to public health programmes may be considered under the headings of health, illness, and treatment behaviours.

### Health behaviour

Health behaviour refers to those activities people undertake to avoid disease and to detect asymptomatic infections through appropriate screening tests. For instance, sexually transmitted disease can be prevented by avoiding sexual exposure with infectious sexual partners. Other health behaviour that might reduce the risks of infection include the use of condoms, of bactericidal products immediately before and after sexual exposure, and the appropriate use of antimicrobial agents with proper supervision (8). In addition, the risks of transmission can be reduced by assisting in the detection of infection in sexual partners before they have further unprotected sexual exposure with other susceptible partners.

People with good health habits (e.g., daily brushing of teeth, routine use of automobile seat-belts, nonsmoking) are less likely to develop venereal infections than persons with poor health habits (9). Sexually active individuals with good health habits are more likely to practise disease prevention and have routine checkups in the absence of symptoms. Therefore, persons with good general health habits need less consideration in programmes designed to improve preventive habits.

In analysing health behaviour with respect to sexually transmitted diseases it is essential to consider the behaviour of sexual partners, not just individuals. An inexperienced female teenager may know that gonorrhoea is spread by sexual intercourse and that it may cause loss of fertility; she may also believe that condoms prevent disease, and may value her reproductive capacity highly. Consequently, she may favour the use of condoms during sexual intercourse. However, unless her infectious boyfriend is also convinced of the value of condoms, they may still have unprotected sexual intercourse. When educational programmes are introduced, they must promote complementary health behaviour in potential sexual partners.

*Illness behaviour*

Illness behaviour refers to how people react to symptoms. Generally, people who detect symptoms will wait to see if the symptoms persist or worsen. If the symptoms continue, the affected person may ask a friend or acquaintance for advice, before seeking medical help. Since the symptoms of sexually transmitted diseases are often mild and transitory, they may not be troublesome enough to encourage the person to seek medical care.

Additional methods of encouraging medical attendance should be sought to increase recognition that genital symptoms may need medical attention. One method is to convert present sufferers from sexually transmitted diseases into advocates for the prompt medical evaluation of all symptomatic persons. One way to encourage this is to ensure that patients are satisfied with the care they have received and, for this reason, the quality of medical care should be improved.

*Treatment behaviour*

Treatment behaviour refers to those activities used to cure diseases and restore health. With reference to sexually transmitted disease, it is particularly important for patients to take the medication as directed, return for tests of cure, and cooperate in efforts to identify untreated sexual partners. Research has not shown that any particular group or personality type is more compliant than any other. Programme managers should develop treatment objectives, implement strategies to enhance appropriate treatment behaviour, and evaluate the results.

## 4.5 Target groups

Sociological concepts of control involve three key groups: influential leaders, technical experts, and priority groups.

Influential leaders must be made aware of the nature and magnitude of the problem of sexually transmitted diseases, its cost to society, and the benefits associated with its prevention and control.

Experts in communications, social, scientific, and medical research exist in most social systems. Programme managers should identify and involve these technical experts in planning and implementing control programmes and collecting new information.

Hosts and susceptibles in the population must be identified and characterized in a way that facilitates effective disease intervention. The value of identifying priority groups for intervention activities has been reviewed (Chapter 3). Programme managers need to develop systematic approaches to these groups to facilitate understanding of the social-cultural settings and to develop more effective ways to work with them.

## References

1. BOGUE, D. J. et al. *Communicating to combat VD*. Chicago, University of Chicago Press, 1979.
2. DARROW, W. W. & PAULI, M. L. Health behaviour and sexually transmitted diseases. In Holmes, K. K. et al., ed. *Sexually transmitted diseases*. New York. McGraw-Hill, 1984.
3. KROGER, F. & WIESNER, P. J. STD education. *Journal of school health*, 51: 242–246 (1981).
4. BECKER, M. H. & MAIMAN, L. A. Sociobehavioral determinants of compliance with health and medical care recommendations. *Medical care*, 13: 10–24 (1975).
5. ROSENTOCK, I. M. Prevention of illness and maintenance of health. In: Kosa, J. et al., ed. *Poverty and health*. Cambridge, MA, Harvard University Press, 1969.
6. DARROW, W. W. *Innovative health behaviour*. Doctoral dissertation. Emory University, Department of Sociology, 1973.
7. ROKEACH, M. *The nature of human values*. New York, Free Press, 1973.
8. DARROW, W. W. Approaches to the problem of venereal disease prevention. *Preventive medicine*, 15:165–175 (1976).
9. DARROW, W. W. Attitudes toward condom use and the acceptance of venereal disease prophylactics. In: Redford, M. H. et al., ed. *The condom: increasing utilization in the United States*. San Francisco, San Francisco Press, 1974.

# PART II

# INTERVENTION STRATEGIES

Intervention strategies are those activities that directly affect the incidence and/or complications of the sexually transmitted disease. Eradication of these diseases could be achieved by the development and mass application of ideal drugs (not currently available) or effective vaccines (not generally available for the organisms involved in sexually transmitted diseases). Conversely, sexual transmission of disease could be eliminated if persons adopted life-long sexual exclusivity between couples. However, sexual exclusivity seems to be decreasing in most countries rather than increasing. Thus, total eradication does not seem to be a feasible programme objective and more limited control objectives are appropriate for most countries.

Intervention strategies are usually aimed at particular groups in the community selected as priorities for intervention. However, control objectives generally refer to reductions in the incidence or associated complications of sexually transmitted diseases as they affect the population as a whole.

Specific aims of intervention strategies are:

(1) to minimize disease exposure by reducing sexual intercourse with persons who have a high probability of being infected;

(2) to prevent infection by increasing the use of condoms or other prophylactic barriers;

(3) to detect and cure disease by implementing disease detection programmes, providing effective diagnostic and treatment facilities, and promoting health-seeking behaviour;

(4) to limit complications of infection by providing early treatment for both symptomatic and asymptomatic infected individuals; and

(5) to limit disease transmission within the community with the above efforts.

The four principal intervention strategies available for the control of sexually transmitted diseases are (1) health promotion (Chapter 5); (2) disease detection (Chapter 6); (3) national treatment programmes (Chapter 7); and (4) contact tracing and patient counselling (Chapter 8). Clinical services (Chapter 9) will be the vehicle for some part of each of these strategies.

Although vaccination strategies for control will become more feasible in the future, vaccines are not yet available for many of the most important sexually transmitted diseases, and those which are currently available are too expensive for use in most control programmes.

# Chapter 5. Health promotion

## 5.1 Introduction

The principal aim of educational intervention is to encourage behaviour which will ultimately reduce the impact of sexually transmitted diseases in the community. Accordingly, the targets for educational efforts may include the general public, patients, priority groups, technical experts, health providers, community leaders, and decision-makers. Comprehensive programmes may aim at all such groups; other educational programmes may select only one or a few groups for directed educational activities.

This chapter outlines an approach to health promotion at the community level. Many methods are considered; their application will vary from country to country.

## 5.2 General principles for designing and implementing educational programmes

*Determination of the specific aims of the programme*

Dissemination of information is not enough. Educational programmes should be designed to enhance individual behaviour related to primary and secondary prevention of disease (i.e., limiting the risk of contracting infection and decreasing the occurrence of complications and further disease transmission once infected). Thus, specific aims of educational intervention may include activities:

(*a*) to promote discriminative sexual intercourse by avoiding multiple and/or casual sexual partners;

(*b*) to promote the use of the condom or other prophylactic methods in at-risk situations;

(*c*) to promote prompt attendance for screening examination after exposure in at-risk situations;

(*d*) to promote early attendance for medical examination when symptomatic;

(*e*) to promote compliance with treatment; and

(*f*) to facilitate other interventions such as referral of sexual partners, treatment compliance, etc.

*Consideration of the sociocultural setting*

Before starting an appropriate programme, relevant characteristics of the community and of the selected target groups must be taken into account (Chapter 3). The customs and beliefs, organization of the social system and the governmental structure or political regime differ from community to community and from one country to another. In addition, the characteristics and organization of the educational target groups vary. Therefore, it may be necessary to have a flexible approach to the educational programme for individual groups and communities.

The control of sexually transmitted diseases poses particular problems for health education. Individual sexual behaviour is often implicated as the sole determinant of infection. Disapproval by the culture of sexual behaviour which leads to disease acquisition may prove a barrier to effective disease control by stigmatizing infected individuals. Thus, all infected individuals may be viewed prejudicially even though their disease was contracted congenitally, or in such blameless ways as from a spouse or a partner who had limited access to care facilities. In addition, the simplistic approach of according individual blame for disease fails to reflect that peer group pressure is a major factor in promoting unhealthy behaviour. Furthermore, messages from the general culture often directly or indirectly promote unhealthy sexual behaviour.

The health action model (Fig. 1) incorporates features of other behavioural models (1–4). It indicates the importance of "drives", as, for example, in the case of an adolescent couple, with a positive attitude to using contraceptives, who have unprotected intercourse under the influence of a more powerful sex "drive." This model also indicates the importance of "facilitating" factors (e.g., peer pressure to engage in sex to demonstrate "maturity") and "inhibiting" factors (e.g., fear of pregnancy). These are the factors that finally influence whether an intended action is translated into actual behaviour.

In order to plan educational strategies most effectively, it is useful to have some understanding of how knowledge, beliefs, attitudes, etc. are acquired during an individual's lifetime (5–7). One approach would be to develop a description of factors influencing disease acquisition throughout life (a "career line" for sexually transmitted disease). This would provide an indication of how parents' attitudes to sexuality, peer pressures during adolescence, and formal sex education programmes at school contribute to the young adult's health and illness behaviour.

It is also important to make an assessment of the organization of the community and to identify influential leaders who could amplify the educational messages. The various community educational resources can also be reviewed to ensure that they are used in a coordinated and cumulative way for maximum effect.

*Selection and preparation of educational messages*

The messages of each programme must take into account the cultural, educational, and economic levels of the community and the specific aims of the programme (e.g., to promote prompt medical examination when symptoms are present and to promote discriminative sexual contact). Messages should be: brief, well-organized, comprehensible to the intended target groups, repetitive, specific (i.e., give instructions on what to do and

Fig. 1. The health action model

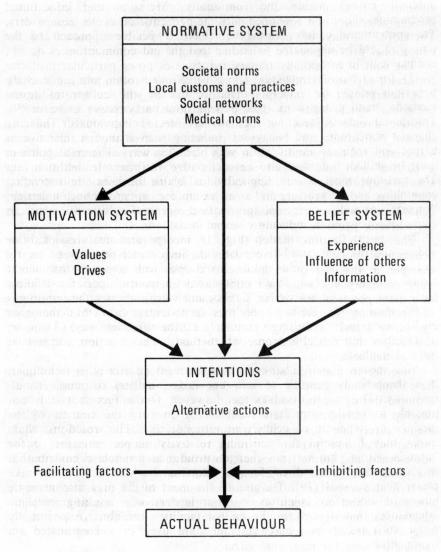

not just generalities), and arranged in order of priority (i.e., the main message should come first) (8). When available, the help of local teachers and communication experts should be sought in order to produce messages with the greatest impact.

*Selection of educational methods*

Detailed information on the communication media is not available in many countries. None the less, it may be possible to estimate the availability of media and to determine their reach, frequency, and penetration of different groups within the community. Messages and educational programmes should be developed with the participation of the local leaders. The content and context should be reviewed with these leaders and the timing should be negotiated to ensure that the education activities do not conflict with important community events.

(1) *Direct teaching methods.* The most effective techniques for teaching behaviour related to sexually transmitted disease will use non-traditional methods: small group work, role playing, and participatory exercises (9). Traditional didactic teaching methods are less appropriate for inducing changes in attitudes and behaviour. Inducing such changes is affective in nature and requires identification with the "teacher." Thus, the teachers must be skilled, but must also have empathy with the intended audience. The methods most widely applicable in health facilities are individual counselling and persuasion, and small group discussions. In such a setting, "experts" providing technical information will be less effective than an empathetic teacher in inducing changes in attitude and behaviour.

To support the information in the discussion sessions, visual aids or audiovisual material can be very helpful. Such materials must be clearly and simply designed, and should avoid technical language that might reduce audience interest. In all presentations a question period will allow participants to raise worries or doubts and clarify areas of uncertainty.

(2) *Mass media.* Research findings consistently show that the mass media, newspapers, radio, television, etc., can be effectively used to support or facilitate other health promotion methods. They are less effective as isolated methods.

Mass media education has one obvious advantage over other techniques: it is theoretically possible to influence large numbers of people simultaneously. The major disadvantage, however, is the fact that it is not possible to obtain immediate feedback or to vary the content of the message or its mode of delivery in response to clients' reactions. Mass media may be useful for providing relatively simple messages or for "agenda setting" but will not change attitudes or promote behaviour that involves undue effort, discomfort, or requires the individual to foresake pleasurable pursuits (10). The use of the mass media may also generate unwanted side-effects such as inappropriate anxiety resulting in clinic attendances that overwhelm the limited facilities available; or potentially worse, such anxiety may make the individual afraid of seeking advice and treatment.

Mass media campaigns will also convince the decision-makers who secured the resources for the programme that it is being carried out.

(3) *Magazines.* Popular magazines provide a potentially valuable source of information on sexually transmitted diseases. Magazine advisers on "life problems" receive large numbers of letters that clearly illustrate the inadequacies of current sex education (11). The use of "girlie" magazines or publications for homosexuals as a way of reaching at-risk groups was viewed favourably in comparative reviews of sexually transmitted disease education in London and New York (12).

The value of comic strips to appeal to at-risk youth should not be ignored. Recent evaluation of comic strips in the context of sex education has been generally favourable (*13*).

(4) *Telephone "hot lines"*. The use of telephone services providing prerecorded messages may sometimes be useful. A telephone service provided in London in the early 1970s received 367 267 calls during a period of 10 months (*14*). In a more recent study in Rotterdam (*15*) 72 536 calls were received during a period of 15 weeks and the authors argued that the system produced an 11 % increase in clinic attendance. Of course, this outcome would be counterproductive unless those attending the clinics had a reasonably high rate of infection. Other telephone services use trained volunteers able to provide information for each individual and appropriate referral alternatives (*16*).

(5) *Other methods and combinations*. It is important to use the wide range of existing media selectively and intelligently and to match the needs of both the teacher and the learner. Alternative media may be effective as adjuncts to other educational strategies. The V.D. Education Unit in New York City reported the effective use of a variety of media: radio messages, bumper stickers for taxis, matchbooks with messages distributed in high-risk localities, a pop record called "Love pollution," and free condom gift certificates (*12*).

Since community readiness and rates of adoption of health messages vary for different population strata, it may be desirable to develop a multimedia approach. The comprehensive, integrated programme in Costa Rica which included newspapers, radio and television messages, audiovisual materials, conferences, posters, and illustrated pamphlets for distribution to schools, colleges, universities, health centres, and hospitals is another example of this approach (*17*). Such a multi-media approach should be used whenever possible.

*Selection of the agents and agencies for health promotion*

Health education and health promotion should be undertaken by agents accepted by the community, such as respected leaders, local teachers, health providers, etc. Education agencies often include:

(1) *The school*. The school can be viewed as the potential primary preventive agency. The differences in school systems both within and between countries will determine whether schools are used to provide health promotion programmes related to the control of sexually transmitted disease. When health agencies and the school collaborate closely in producing coherent health education programmes, the results can be most satisfactory.

(2) *Medical services*. Whether the services specific for sexually transmitted diseases are provided in specialist clinics or at the primary care level, it is essential that all personnel who have patient contact, such as clinicians, auxiliary staff, social workers, and receptionists, are involved in the educational effort. Such personnel may need additional training to enable

them to fulfil their role as teachers. In addition to the educational, counselling and social-interaction skills and techniques which must be mastered, the personnel must also be encouraged to adopt a positive attitude towards their education duties.

(3) *Others.* Direct educational messages may be conveyed by other influential leaders or agents in the community. The impact of educational activities largely depends on the personal characteristics of the teacher. If the teacher appears to have several characteristics in common with those at whom the message is directed such as social status, ethnic or religious background, then he or she is more likely to be influential (*18*). However, those lacking such common characteristics may still be influential if they are sympathetic and understanding in their approach.

### Development of community outreach activities

Outreach programmes ensure that the whole population receives the educational message and not merely the better-educated, urban populations. This is especially important since there are many problems associated with sexually transmitted diseases in the rural or peri-urban populations of developing countries and amongst the disadvantaged urban populations in industrialized nations. The use of community development and "outreach" programmes has achieved success in many health fields (*19*). For example, volunteer peer counsellors in the London "Grapevine" project successfully contacted young people—many of whom could not be contacted through more formal "establishment" approaches (*20*).

### Community participation

Active participation by the community throughout the design and implementation of a health programme is vital to its success. This principle is particularly relevant to health promotion programmes for sexually transmitted disease. A motivated, actively-involved population may help by identifying venues for particularly relevant activities and by providing financial resources or helpers. For full impact, leaders of community opinion must be encouraged to participate and to become spokesmen for health promotion.

### Integration of education with other health programmes

Education programmes for sexually transmitted diseases may have the greatest impact when they are an integral part of other programmes. Health programmes which may be particularly relevant include family planning, mental health, drug programmes, mother–child organizations, general community-based programmes, and programmes for juveniles. Incorporating education on the subject of sexually transmitted disease into these other programmes ensures that the topic is covered and may also facilitate its acceptance. However, care must be taken in the design and presentation of such integrated health education programmes so that the specific educational messages are not obscured or ignored.

## 5.3 Evaluation

Evaluation is an essential component of any strategy or programme (Chapter 15). The process of evaluation may measure changes in disease prevalence or incidence, but more typically involves shorter-term measures such as changes in behaviour (e.g., compliance); changes in knowledge, beliefs, or attitudes; or the acquisition of new skills. Such measures must be assessed depending upon the way in which the changes relate to other variables and to the ultimate behaviour of individuals.

Evaluation will measure the extent to which behavioural objectives have been achieved, and it may be used as a basis for securing further resources for the control programme. More directly, however, evaluation allows the identification of performance problems that can lead to programme modifications, which will make the programme more effective.

## References

1. BECKER, M. H., ed. *The health belief model and personal health behavior*. Thorofare, NJ, Charles B. Slack, 1974.
2. BARIC, L. Non-smokers, smokers, ex-smokers: Three separate problems for health education. *International journal of health education*, **22**: (1 Supplement). 1–20 (1979).
3. FREIDSON, E. Client control and medical behaviour. *American journal of sociology*, **65**: 377 (1960).
4. FISHBEIN, M. & AJZEN, I. *Belief, attitude, intention and behaviour: An introduction to theory and research*. New York, Addison and Wesley, 1975.
5. TONES, B. K. Socialisation, health career and the health education of the schoolchild. *Journal of the Institute of Health Education*, **15**: 22–29 (1977).
6. THORNBURG, H. D. Adolescent sources of information on sex. *School health*, **51**: 274–278 (1981).
7. SCHOFIELD, M. *The sexual behaviour of young adults*. London, Allen Lane, 1973.
8. GREEN, L. W. Education strategies to improve compliance with therapeutic and preventive regimens: the recent evidence. In: *Compliance in health care*. Baltimore-London, The Johns Hopkins University Press, 1979.
9. SNEGROFF, S. Venereal disease education: facts are not enough. *School health*, **45**: 37–39 (1975).
10. TONES, B. K. The use and abuse of mass media in health promotion. In: Leathar, D. S. et al., ed. *Health education and the media*. Oxford, Pergamon Press, 1981.
11. PROOPS, M. The journalists point of view. In: *Sex education of schoolchildren*. London, Royal Society for Health, 1971.
12. GOOSEY, R. S.T.D. A comparative study: New York–England. Diploma dissertation, Leeds Polytechnic, Leeds, England, 1978.
13. CURTIS, S. *Don't rush me. The comic-strip, sex education and a multi-racial society*. London, Community Relations Commission, 1975.
14. *The control of the spread of gonorrhoea: A health education exercise to improve contact tracing. Final report to Health Education Council*. London, 1975.
15. SCHUURMAN, J. & DE HAES, W. Sexually transmitted diseases: Health education by telephone. *International journal of health education*, **23** No. 2: 94–106 (1980).
16. KNOX, S. R. ET AL. Profile of callers to the VD national hotline. *Sexually transmitted diseases*, **8**: 245–254 (1981).

17. JARAMILLO, O. ET AL. Costa Rica: Programa para el control de las enfermedades de transmisión sexual. *Boletín de la Oficina sanitaria panamericana*, **86**: 131–140 (1979).
18. ROGERS, E. M. & SHOEMAKER, F. F. *The communication of innovations*. New York, The Free Press, 1971.
19. SIMMONS, J. ed. *Making health education work*. Washington, DC, American Public Health Association, 1976.
20. GRAPEVINE COMMUNITY SEX EDUCATION PROJECT. *Report on the experimental period ending 30 November 1974*. Grapevine, 296 Holloway Road, London N. 7.

# Chapter 6. Disease detection

## 6.1 Introduction

Disease detection is an essential part of any control programme. The identification of infected individuals combined with rapid treatment will reduce the complications of disease and minimize further transmission of disease in the community (*1*). In some circumstances screening and case-finding activities may be the first feasible step in a population-based control programme for sexually transmitted disease. For example, the prevention of the effects of syphilis on pregnancy through antenatal case-finding may be selected as the initial priority of a control programme. Screening and case-finding activities also allow for a better understanding of the nature and magnitude of the disease problem in a particular setting.

This chapter deals with tests and activities related to screening and case-finding programmes, collectively referred to as early disease detection programmes.

## 6.2 Definitions

*Diagnosis*

Diagnosis of disease in patients who have sought health care involves a variety of questions, examinations, and tests; in this way the exact cause of their complaint can be established. Early diagnosis (and treatment) is extremely important and is determined largely by the quality and quantity of available services (Chapter 9).

*Epidemiological surveys*

Epidemiological surveys involve the measurement of demographic, social, behavioural, and biological characteristics of samples of carefully selected populations during cross-sectional or prevalence studies. Because the main objective of the survey is to acquire new knowledge, no direct health benefit to the participants is implied, even though persons found to have a problem are usually referred for treatment. Surveys indirectly affect health; for example by describing the magnitude of the problem in a community, epidemiological surveys may lead to more effective control programmes (Chapter 2).

Epidemiological surveys to determine the prevalence of the disease, or of risk factors associated with disease, have most often been used for the chronic, non-infectious diseases of advanced age (coronary heart disease, chronic lung disease, hypertension, etc.) (*2*). Epidemiological surveys of sexually transmitted diseases in large representative groups of the population have rarely been done, exceptions being a recent surveys conducted in the United Kingdom (3) and the relevant parts of the periodic surveys carried out by the National Center for Health Statistics in the United States of America (4).

Surveys of disease prevalence have been conducted frequently in selected population groups known or suspected to be at high risk such as prostitutes (5, 6) and homosexuals (7). Such small-scale surveys can provide baseline data for considering control measures, particularly screening, for these groups.

*Screening*

Screening is the testing, not of carefully selected population samples, but of apparently healthy volunteers from the general population for the purpose of separating them into groups with high and low probabilities of contracting a given disorder. As in the epidemiological survey, the encounter is initiated by those who do the tests; the objective is the early detection (and treatment) of disease, with the implicit premise that volunteers will benefit from the screening programme. An example of screening for a sexually transmitted disease is serological testing for syphilis in military recruits or personal service workers.

Early detection tests are carried out in many countries. Most of these programmes are called "screening" but in fact are based on the case-finding principle (see below). Although the distinction between these two methods may be conceptually important, both may detect disease and may be useful for disease control. In many settings the term "screening" is still used to refer to both screening and case-finding activities.

*Case-finding*

Case-finding is a form of disease detection in which individuals seeking health care for any reason are given additional tests to detect sexually transmitted disease. A traditional example is serological testing for syphilis of adult patients admitted to hospitals. As such, case-finding could be considered an extension of the clinical evaluation during a patient-generated encounter.

**6.3 Properties of tests used in early detection programmes**

Early detection usually depends upon laboratory tests. The properties of the tests and the programmes which use them are extensively discussed in epidemiological textbooks (8, 9). These can be summarized as follows (see also reference 2):

(a) *Accuracy*: ability to give a true measurement of the item being tested.

(b) *Precision*: reproducibility in repeated trials. Precision is affected by the variation inherent in the method, and the observer variation (10).

(c) *Sensitivity*: ability of the test to give a positive result when the individual tested has the disease.

(d) *Specificity*: ability of the test to give a negative result when the individual tested is free of the disease.

(e) *Validity*: the extent to which individuals are rightly identified as having or not having the disease. Validity is thus a function of the sensitivity and specificity of a test.

(f) *Simplicity*: ease of test performance.

(g) *Predictive value*: the extent to which a positive test correctly identifies a person with disease, also referred to as Bayes' theorem. While validity is an abstract rating of the test, the predictive value describes the operational performance of the test within a population that has a particular disease prevalence. When prevalence of the disease is low, even a highly specific test gives a relatively large number of false positives owing to the many non-infected individuals being tested.

Table 3 shows the predictive values of a positive test with constant and high validity, at two levels of disease prevalence, 1% and 20%. When disease prevalence is low, that is 1%, the positive predictive value of this highly valid test is 17%; in other words, 5 out of 6 individuals who have a positive test do not have the disease. The predictive value increases rapidly with increasing disease prevalence so that at 20% prevalence, the predictive value of a positive test is 83%, i.e., 83% of persons with a positive test have the disease.

(h) *Yield*: the amount of previously unrecognized disease that is diagnosed as a result of the early detection effort. Yield depends on many factors including the sensitivity of the test, prevalence of the disease, extent of other screening, and the participation of individuals in the detection effort. The yield or true discovery rate of the early detection programme can be distinguished from those discoveries that merely validate a diagnosis

Table 3. Predictive values of a positive test with 99% specificity at two levels of prevalence

|  | Prevalence | |
|---|---|---|
|  | 1% | 20% |
| (a) Number in population | 1000 | 1000 |
| (b) Diseased | 10 | 200 |
| (c) Non-diseased | 990 | 800 |
| (d) True positives (b ×0.99) | 10 (9.9) | 198 |
| (e) False positives (c ×[1–0.95]) | 50 (49.5) | 40 |
| (f) Total positives (d + e) | 60 | 238 |
| (g) Predictive values of positive test (d/f) | $\frac{10}{60} = 17\%$ | $\frac{198}{238} = 83\%$ |

in a patient who already received treatment on clinical as well as on epidemiological grounds.

## 6.4 Principles of early detection of disease

Some basic principles proposed for large-scale screening programmes for chronic disease (12–15) should be considered when formulating an early detection programme for sexually transmitted diseases: (a) the condition sought should be an important health problem; (b) there should be an accepted treatment for patients with recognized disease; (c) facilities for diagnosis and treatment should be available; (d) there should be a recognizable latent or early symptomatic stage; (e) there should be a suitable test or examination; (f) the test should be acceptable to the population (in terms of discomfort, time, etc.); (g) the natural history of the condition, including development from latent to overt disease, should be adequately understood; (h) the cost of case-finding (including diagnosis and treatment of patient diagnosed) should be economically balanced in relation to total possible expenditure on medical care; and (i) case-finding should be a continuing process and not a "once and for all" project.

## 6.5 Other considerations for early detection programmes

### Target population

Before deciding on an early detection programme, the group to be screened must be considered further. What population should be screened in order to maximize the health benefits of such a control effort? This will depend upon the focus of the control programme and the intervention efforts. Will the activities have other positive or negative effects on the screened population? Thus, disease detection may further stigmatize some population groups, e.g., prostitutes; alternatively, identification of disease in pregnant women, for example, may help to emphasize that sexually transmitted diseases can occur in any group thereby helping to destigmatize these diseases. Finally, if early disease detection increases the population's anxiety, demand for health services may suddenly increase.

### Future and scope of the programme

When an early detection programme that has been successful during pilot studies is expanded into a large-scale programme, difficulties will be encountered and resource needs will be sizeable. But more importantly, when moving from essentially a small research investigation depending on a limited number of motivated persons to a routine every-day practice, the problems of implementation and of ensuring the continued quality of the project may be substantial.

## 6.6 Experiences with screening and case-finding programmes

*Prevalence of disease*

The decision to initiate, continue, or abandon a screening programme is often determined by the prevalence of the disease in the population being screened. In many industrialized countries the prevalence of syphilis has become so low that the cost-effectiveness of serological screening and systematic case-finding (e.g., in premarital examinations, prenatal examinations, and examinations of new admissions to hospitals or clinics) is being questioned (*16, 17*). Similarly, mass case-finding programmes for gonorrhoea in women were not implemented in European countries owing to the low prevalence of the disease (*3*).

The prevalence of disease also affects the predictive value of test results. For example, the Wassermann test is known to give at least 0.03% false positives (30 false positives in 100 000 tests) (*18, 19*). In 1940, the prevalence of syphilis among draft examinees in the USA was 4530 per 100 000 and in 1977 it fell to 180 per 100 000; this results in a predictive value of a positive Wassermann test of 99.3% in 1940 and of 85.7% in 1977, respectively. The prevalence of syphilis in new blood donors in Belgium has been reported to be 25 per 100 000; therefore, the predictive value of a Wassermann test should be 45% in Belgium (*20*).

*Impact of early detection programmes*

The United States of America initiated a massive gonorrhoea case-finding programme in 1972, using cervical cultures as part of an overall control programme aimed at changing the incidence of gonorrhoea (*21–24*). Up to nine million cultures were performed per year, of which 4.5% were positive. The effect of this large-scale programme has been difficult to evaluate. Using an epidemiological model, it was concluded that the programme seems to have held the incidence of gonorrhoea at an equilibrium 20% below that which would exist without the programme (*25*). In addition, reported incidence rates of gonorrhoea declined 6% from 1975 to 1980 (*26*). Of course, other factors could have been responsible for the changes in incidence, such as more adequate treatment based on effective treatment recommendations, improved sexual partner referral efforts, etc. Visits to doctors for acute pelvic inflammatory disease also decreased following the gonorrhoea case-finding programme, but methodological problems limit the evaluation of this effect (*27*).

*Yield and cost of programmes*

Yield and cost considerations may be particularly important in screening or case-finding activities; selection of the target population may greatly influence these factors. During the gonorrhoea programmes (see above), the cost per case detected varied from US$25.00 in metropolitan venereal disease clinics to US$350.00 in areas of low prevalence (*21*). When more selective case-finding was instituted in one programme in 1976, the proportion of positive tests increased from 4.5 % to 8.1 % in one year, and the cost per case detected was considerably reduced (22).

Screening has been considered in some high-risk groups such as homosexuals and prostitutes. In many countries Gram stains for gonorrhoea are used in the compulsory screening of legalized or semi-legalized prostitutes. The yields are usually low (28) and the impact is probably only indirect, i.e., prostitutes become more careful, more hygienic, seek medical care earlier, or otherwise treat themselves. The usefulness of such compulsory screening with Gram stains is still a debatable issue.

Another group at high-risk of infection which has been proposed as a target population for future screening is present sufferers from a sexually transmitted disease. In one study, in which former patients were re-evaluated after a period of several weeks, the cost of detecting a new case of gonorrhoea was shown to be US$ 796.00 (21). This particular screening activity was not considered cost-effective in the setting where it was evaluated.

*Early detection and case management*

If early disease detection is to influence disease control, the infected individuals detected by the programme must receive further management. A major problem contributing to the poor cost-effectiveness of screening or case-finding for sexually transmitted disease is the low follow-up rate of the positive cases detected. The prevalence of gonorrhoea in family planning acceptors in Johannesburg was 10.2 %, but only 46 % of the positive cases could be treated (29). In Salisbury (now Harare, Zimbabwe), the prevalence of gonorrhoea was 2 % in pregnant women, 11 % in gynaecological patients, and 12 % in family planning patients, but 3 months after these cases were detected only 30 % of the positive cases had been treated (30).

## 6.7 Conclusions

Screening and case-finding activities define only one aspect of disease morbidity and that is prevalence. Prevalence depends both on the incidence of the disease and on its duration. Thus, infections of longer duration can be easily identified by disease detection programmes. These infections include asymptomatic gonococcal or chlamydial genital infections, latent syphilis, and carriers of hepatitis B. When early detection programmes are introduced, facilities for further diagnosis and treatment must be available.

The selection of both the target population and the type of detection programme should be dictated by the type and importance of the particular problem, and the cost and technical feasibility of the intervention.

Early detection directly influences the duration of infection. Thus, the main health benefits may be fewer complications in the individual and his/her offspring. Such detection programmes will reduce disease transmission and incidence only if the cases discovered are "transmitters" of disease.

## References

1. HART, G. Screening to control infectious diseases. Evaluation of control programs for gonorrhoea and syphilis. *Reviews of infectious diseases,* **2**: 701–712 (1980).
2. SACKETT, D. L. & HOLLAND, W. W. Controversy in the detection of disease. *Lancet,* **2**: 357–359 (1975).
3. ADLER, M. W. ET AL. Sexually transmitted diseases in a defined population of women. *British medical journal,* **283**: 29–32 (1981).
4. NATIONAL CENTRE FOR HEALTH STATISTICS. *Plan and operation of the second national health and nutrition survey 1976–80.* Hyattsville, MD, NCHS, 1981 (*Vital and health statistics,* Series 1. No. 15—DHHS publication no. (PHS 81–1317).
5. MEHEUS, A. ET AL. Prevalence of gonorrhoea in prostitutes in a Central African town. *British journal of venereal diseases,* 50–52 (1974).
6. POTTERAT, J. J. ET AL. Gonorrhoea in street prostitutes. *Sexually transmitted diseases,* **6**: 58–63 (1979).
7. BLEEKER, A. ET AL. Prevalence of syphilis and hepatitis B among homosexual men in two saunas in Amsterdam. *British journal of venereal diseases,* **57**: 196–199 (1981).
8. MACMAHON, B. & PUGH, T. F. *Epidemiology: Principles and methods.* Boston, Little Brown, 1970.
9. MAUSNER, J. S. & BAHN, A. K. *Epidemiology – an introductory text.* Philadelphia, Saunders Co., 1974.
10. WILLCOX, J. R. ET AL. Observer variation in the interpretation of Gram-stained urethral smears – implications for the diagnosis of non-specific urethritis. *British journal of venereal diseases,* **57**: 134–136 (1981).
11. ARMITAGE, P. *Statistical methods in medical research.* Oxford, Blackwell Scientific Publications, 1973.
12. WILSON, J. M. G. & JUNGNER, G. *Principles and practice of screening for disease.* Geneva, World Health Organization, 1968 (Public Health Papers No. 34).
13. MCKEOWN, T. ed. *Screening in medical care: reviewing the evidence.* London, Oxford University Press, 1968.
14. COCHRANE, A. L. & HOLLAND, W. W. Validation of screening procedures. *British medical bulletin,* **27**: 3–8 (1971).
15. WHITBY, G. L. Screening for disease, definition and criteria. *Lancet,* **2**: 819–821 (1974).
16. FELMAN, Y. M. Repeal of mandated premarital tests for syphilis: A survey of State health officers. *American journal of public health,* **71**: 155–159 (1981).
17. KINGON, R. J. & WIESNER, P. J. Premarital syphilis screening: Weighing the benefits. *American journal of public health,* **71**: 160–162 (1981).
18. TRAMONT, E. C. *Treponema pallidum* (syphilis). In: Mandell, G. L. et al., ed. *Principles and practice of infectious diseases.* New York, John Wiley & Sons, 1979.
19. MACFARLANE, D. E. & ELIAS-JONES, T. F. Screening tests for syphilis. A comparison of the Treponema Pallidum Haemagglutination Assay with two automated serological tests. *British journal of venereal diseases,* **53**: 348–352 (1977).
20. MEHEUS, A. Prevalence studies. In: Holland, W. W. & Karhausen, L., ed. *Health care and epidemiology.* London, Kimpton Publishers, 1978.
21. ST. JOHN, R. K. & CURRAN, J. W. Epidemiology of gonorrhoea. *Sexually transmitted diseases,* **6**: 81–82 (1978).
22. FELMAN, Y. M. ET AL. Gonorrhoea screening. Experience of a large municipal program. *New York State journal of medicine,* **78**: 1267–1270 (1978).
23. HINMAN, A. R. Prevention and control of gonorrhoea in the United States. In: Robert, R. B., ed. *The gonococcus.* New York, John Wiley & Sons, 1977.
24. HENDERSON, R. H. Control of sexually transmitted diseases in the United States. A federal perspective. *British journal of venereal diseases,* **53**: 211–215 (1977).
25. YORKE, J. A. ET AL. Dynamics and control of the transmission of gonorrhoea. *Sexually transmitted diseases,* **5**: 51–56 (1978).

26. CENTERS FOR DISEASE CONTROL. Sexually transmitted diseases. Statistical Letter, 1980, CDC, Atlanta, 1982.
27. CENTERS FOR DISEASE CONTROL. Pelvic inflammatory disease-United States. *Morbidity and mortality weekly report*, **28**: 605–607 (1980).
28. REEVES, W. C. ET AL. Epidemiología de las enfermedades trasmitidas sexualmente en un grupe de mujeres de alto riesgo en Panamá. *Revista médica de Panamá*, **5**: 209–222 (1980).
29. HALL, S. M. & WHITCOMB, M. A. Screening for gonorrhoea in family planning acceptors in a developing community. *Public health (London)*, **92**: 121–124 (1978).
30. WEISSENBERG, R. ET AL. The incidence of gonorrhoea in urban Rhodesian black women. *South African medical journal*, **57**: 1119–1120 (1977).

# Chapter 7. National treatment programmes

## 7.1 Introduction

Early and adequate treatment of patients and their sexual partners is an effective way of preventing the trend of increasing antimicrobial resistance to the microorganisms which cause sexually transmitted diseases, the spread of these diseases, and the development of serious sequelae in individual patients. Barriers to the implementation of this strategy include: the inability of treatment providers to identify infected persons, the selection of ineffective treatment regimens, and the unavailability of treatment for many patients and their sexual partners.

National treatment recommendations are a fundamental part of the process of developing a national treatment programme. However, to have a substantial effect on disease control, the recommended treatments must be used by a large number of those who provide treatment. Unless it is ensured that the treatment recommendations are understood and used, they will not contribute to disease control.

## 7.2 Principles

### Identification and involvement of key decision-makers

The involvement of numerous decision-makers in the development of a national treatment programme will facilitate the subsequent implementation of the programme. These people will need to influence the treatment providers and mobilize the resources required.

### Definition of the problem

The magnitude of the treatment problem must be assessed, and the proportion of the problem that results from the use of ineffective drug regimens or the non-availability of treatment must be established. It will also be useful to identify the reasons why different treatment providers use ineffective treatments. Other information may clarify how the treatment problems contribute to the overall problems caused by sexually transmitted diseases; for example, widespread use of ineffective therapy may select for progressively more resistant microorganisms.

### Development of a plan

After establishing the treatment problems faced by a particular programme, a plan should be drawn up outlining a treatment programme.

41

The coordinated effort of many groups is essential to the success of the programme. The plan should also allow for the evaluation of the programme to identify those areas where full programme implementation has occurred and to relate these successes to any change in the incidence of disease. In addition, the evaluation process can identify remaining problems of implementation and help to find ways to overcome these problems.

## 7.3 National treatment recommendations

One successful approach to the development of a national treatment programme is to develop standard treatment recommendations and use them to define acceptable, effective treatment practices. Other more direct methods should also be considered for different settings, for example, adopting recommendations from elsewhere and passing these directly to treatment providers through a programme of visits.

*Five principles involved in the establishment of treatment recommendations*

(1) *A group of experts should consider the available data about treatment.* Developments in the field have rapidly modified the information used to make decisions concerning the treatment for sexually transmitted diseases. Consequently, health care practices for these diseases are frequently outmoded or haphazard. Health care providers require the assistance of such an expert group to review the latest data and to integrate this into a coherent treatment strategy.

(2) *Simple, direct approaches to diagnosis and treatment may be more feasible and more effective than more sophisticated or complex methods.* Individual articles, chapters, or books tend to recommend treatment only after a specific microbiological etiology has been demonstrated. They also tend to recommend sophisticated, expensive regimens for treatment. When a number of experts review this area, they can make recommendations that are both practical and feasible.

(3) *Treatment standards must be appropriate to the background and setting of the health care providers for whom they are intended.* Infected patients are treated by a wide variety of health care personnel. Those who set the standards must be familiar with the capabilities of the health care personnel who treat the majority of patients in order to produce appropriate recommendations.

(4) *Epidemiological treatment should be encouraged and standardized.* Disease control can be improved by the use of full therapeutic dose treatment for selected groups of individuals before the infection is specifically identified by laboratory tests. Such groups include those who are sexual partners of patients already suffering from a sexually transmitted disease.

(5) *Optimal treatment recommendations transferred from one setting to another cannot necessarily be expected to be appropriate to the new situation.* This transfer of an "ideal" therapy will not be successful unless the

resources, availability of drugs, types of health personnel administering the drugs, susceptibility of microorganisms, and the capability of the recommending officials to influence actual practice are all similar. Care should be taken in selecting experts to ensure that they are familiar with the country and its clinical practices. They should be encouraged to consider a wide range of options.

*Specific methodology*

(1) *Selection of experts.* Selected experts should represent a variety of disciplines (venereology, preventive medicine, primary care, epidemiology, clinical specialties, microbiology), and public and private health officials. They may be assisted by experts from outside the country. The persons selected should be of sufficient academic, scientific, or administrative stature to lend credibility to the recommendations.

Careful consideration should also be given to the personal characteristics of the expert panel. Since a strict quantitative analysis of the treatment problem is not usually possible, the collective judgement of a panel of experts assumes great importance. Thus, authoritarian experts should not be selected, so that dynamic group discussion can occur. Likewise, it is important to select individuals and groups that will aid in the dissemination of the recommendations after they have been established.

(2) *Steps prior to a meeting of experts.* Organization of the available data beforehand is absolutely essential to the success of the meeting. Reviews undertaken by other national public health groups (*1–3*) or by the World Health Organization can provide relevant reference material (*4–8*). Any reports by national investigators should be added to the reviews mentioned.

An adequate overview of the problem of sexually transmitted disease should emphasize those areas where treatment standards are most important. Recommendations can initially be limited to the most common diseases which have the most serious consequences and can be treated. It is also preferable to draft the recommendations so that they will remain appropriate for a substantial period of time. In summary, recommendations should be of limited scope and feasible. Such recommendations can be modified in the future as changes occur.

(3) *Expert group meeting.* The expert group will need to consider initially which individuals should receive treatment. In general, patients should be treated when their probability of having infection is sufficiently high to justify the risks and costs of the treatment. Such treatment criteria must be separated from the diagnostic criteria used for the surveillance of disease trends.

The criteria used to define treatment needs may involve a variety of parameters (Table 4). The expert group must consider which criteria are appropriate for their setting and for the particular care providers within that setting. If many care providers do not have access to diagnostic tests, treatment recommendations may have to be made for clinical syndromes,

## Table 4.  Possible criteria to define persons in need of treatment

(1) *Demographic or geographical criteria*
   high risk for disease defined on the basis of age, race or ethnic group, place of residence, occupation, etc.

(2) *Exposure criteria*
   high risk for disease defined on the basis of sexual exposure to an infected individual

(3) *Clinical criteria*
   high risk for disease defined on the basis of symptoms and/or signs

(4) *Laboratory criteria*
   high risk for disease defined on the basis of microscopical, serological, or culture tests

e.g., urethral discharge or genital ulcer disease. Such recommendations will need to encompass common etiologies of these conditions.

(4) *Regimen characteristics.* On the basis of the preliminary literature survey, the experts should develop an inclusive list of efficacious drug regimens for consideration. The appropriateness of each potential drug regimen should then be evaluated. This process will often result in the reordering of the most appropriate treatments. The characteristics of potential treatment regimens to be considered are: availability, convenience, effectiveness, cost, and possible side-effects. The availability of drugs is influenced by manufacturing and marketing practices, health regulations, and distribution systems. If a drug is simply unobtainable, it should not appear on the treatment recommendations until it becomes available.

The convenience of a drug regimen is an extremely important practical consideration to be taken into account. For instance, oral single-dose regimens are generally more convenient to dispense than parenteral or multiple-dose regimens. Other aspects of convenience which also affect the utilization of a regimen include storage requirements, packaging, and equipment needed to administer the drug.

The effectiveness of a regimen is a very complex issue encompassing compliance, achievable serum levels, susceptibility of the organism, and other factors. Multiple-day regimens may be less effective in practice than in clinical studies because of problems of patient compliance. The susceptibility of the infecting organism is probably the single most important variable. Tremendous geographical variation in antimicrobial susceptibility patterns exist for the gonococcus and probably also for other causative organisms (9, 10). (The syphilis spirochaete is a notable exception; no variation in antimicrobial susceptibility has been identified.)

Consequently, reports of regimen efficacy can be useful only when they originate from countries with similar antimicrobial susceptibility patterns. For example, gonorrhoea treatment regimens that are effective in European countries are often less useful in African countries and of little use in many Asian countries. Weight, gastrointestinal or intramuscular absorption of the drug, and other health status factors may influence the serum level of the drug and thereby determine its effectiveness. Another important aspect of effectiveness arises from the fact that patients often have simultaneous infections of two or more sexually transmitted diseases. Drug regimens that are effective against commonly coexisting infections, e.g., gonorrhoea and chlamydia, will be preferred to those regimens which treat only one infection (*11*).

The cost of a regimen will always be an important consideration. Since the bulk purchase of drugs may reduce costs, the figures used must reflect the actual charges made to programmes or patients. Drug costs should include the equipment, facilities and personnel needed to administer the drugs, and also the cost of the system to procure, store, and distribute the drugs.

The side-effects of regimens also influence the choice of drugs. Both serious life-threatening or permanent adverse effects as well as more frequent, bothersome side-effects need to be considered. Each type of side-effect will have implications for the treatment programme (e.g., gastro-intestinal symptoms of some multiple-day antibiotic regimens may decrease compliance).

Once each regimen has been carefully characterized, a judgement should be made about which regimens are the most appropriate for various groups of patients. The groups will include adults in general and special groups such as pregnant women, allergic patients, children, newborn infants, and sexual partners. For example, pregnant women and young children should not receive tetracycline treatment; and only very safe drugs should be used to treat sexual partners.

(5) *Preparation of the recommendations.* Treatment recommendations should be brief and specific, and any detailed discussion should be reserved for background papers which can be made available upon request. Before the recommendations are finalized, they should be widely circulated for review and comment, and the expert group should then incorporate any relevant changes.

(6) *Dissemination of the recommendations.* The most effective means of disseminating the final recommendations will depend upon the prevailing health care and political system, and the organization of medical education within the country. Existing educational structures should be used initially before new ones are created. It is best to channel the recommendations toward those medical groups, health care organizations, and health care providers treating large numbers of patients. The recommendations should be published in journals and government publications, and also be incorporated into continuing medical education courses. Other methods of dissemination unique to an individual country should be exploited.

## 7.4 Implementation

Whatever methods are used to establish a treatment programme, its implementation requires the maximum support of treatment providers. Such providers need to be trained to use the appropriate regimens for the important sexually transmitted diseases. The resources necessary to ensure their training must be made available. In addition, they must have access to the required drugs in adequate quantities.

## 7.5 Evaluation

The implementation plan should incorporate methods to evaluate both the process and the outcome of the treatment programme. Thus, it will be essential to evaluate periodically the degree to which the information has reached the target population of providers and whether the providers have used the treatments. Overall evaluation of the impact of the programme will be more difficult. However, the effect of the programme on antimicrobial susceptibility patterns can be assessed directly using periodic surveys.

## References

1. CENTERS FOR DISEASE CONTROL. Syphilotherapy, 1976. *Journal of the American Venereal Disease Association*, **3**: 98–180 (1976).
2. CENTERS FOR DISEASE CONTROL. Gonorrhea therapy, *Sexually transmitted diseases*, **6**: 87–194 (1979).
3. CENTERS FOR DISEASE CONTROL. Sexually transmitted diseases therapy, 1982. *Review of infectious diseases*. **4**: 727–890 (1982).
4. IDSOE, O. ET AL. Penicillin in the treatment of syphilis. *Bulletin of the World Health Organization*, **47** (Suppl): 1–68 (1972).
5. WHO Technical Report Series, No. 616, 1976 (Neisseria gonorrhoeae *and gonococcal infections*: report of a WHO Scientific Group).
6. WHO Technical Report Series, No. 660, 1980 (*Nongonococcal urethritis and other sexually transmitted infections of public health importance*: report of a WHO Scientific Group).
7. WHO Technical Report Series, No. 674, 1982 (*Treponemal infections*: report of a WHO Scientific Group).
8. WILLCOX, R. R. *Guide to the management of sexually transmitted infections for general practitioners*. Copenhagen, World Health Organization Regional Office for Europe, 1978.
9. Global distribution of β-lactamase-producing *Neisseria gonorrhoeae*. *Epidemiological bulletin. Pan American Health Organization*, **2** (4): 8–9 (1981).
10. BROWN, S. T. ET AL., Antimicrobial resistance of *Neisseria gonorrhoeae* in Bangkok: Is single drug treatment passé? *Lancet*, **2**: 1366–1368 (1982).
11. WASHINGTON, A. E. Update on treatment recommendations for gonococcal infections. *Reviews of infectious diseases*, **4**: 758–771 (1982).

# Chapter 8. Contact tracing and patient counselling

## 8.1 Introduction

Traditionally, control programmes for sexually transmitted diseases have assumed that patients play relatively passive roles in disease control and prevention. Efforts to identify and treat the sexual partners of infected patients, therefore, involve the health provider interviewing the patient, locating the named individuals and ensuring that these individuals are examined and treated (*1*). This process, generally known as contact tracing, often involves the active participation of the patient. Instead of relying solely on the health worker, the patient may now be encouraged to assume responsibility for locating and referring his or her sexual partners.

The traditional object of contact tracing, to ensure that sexual partners are examined, has been expanded in an effort to change the patients' behaviour which affects acquisition and transmission of disease, compliance with disease management, and other health and illness behaviours (*2*). This behaviour includes (*a*) promptly seeking appropriate medical help in response to the first symptoms, (*b*) taking medication as directed, (*c*) returning for follow-up tests, (*d*) assuring the examination of sexual partners, (*e*) reducing transmission by avoiding exposure until a follow-up test is performed or while symptoms are present, and (*f*) by using protection in high-risk settings.

This chapter discusses contact tracing because this activity is a part of control programmes in many different settings. Although its effectiveness is not questioned, its cost and feasibility for many settings or many subpopulations must be carefully evaluated by programme managers. However, even in cases of apparent failure, and before this preventive measure is withdrawn, it is essential to ensure that any apparent ineffectiveness of contact tracing is not the result of poor performance by those responsible for this activity.

## 8.2 Types of contact tracing

*Formal contact tracing*

This is a system in which specially trained staff interview patients, obtain names and addresses of sexual partners, locate these partners, and offer them examination and treatment. The major objective of formal contact tracing is to reduce disease transmission by locating the individual who was the *source* of the patient's infection. During this process, other persons to whom the disease may have been spread will be identified, thus reducing subsequent disease transmission and complications.

It is generally unproductive to use formal contact tracing where sound diagnostic procedures are not used. Thus, contact tracing is not indicated for patients without disease or with non-infectious disease (e.g., late syphilis). Contact tracing is also less productive with patients whose sexual partners are anonymous, e.g., prostitutes and some homosexuals, or if there are long delays (months) before the sexual partners can be located, e.g., nomadic populations or international travellers.

Other considerations affecting the use of this method include the cost, since this is an expensive form of disease prevention. Thus, comparisons must be made with other aspects of the overall disease control since scarce resources devoted to contact tracing may have to be diverted from other activities, including surveillance, screening, diagnosis, treatment, and education. In addition, even when experienced interviewers are readily available, they may be more usefully employed in another area of the programme. For example, such personnel might be used to elicit information about the dynamics of disease dissemination with members of priority groups. Such information can then be used as the basis for developing new interventions which would be both acceptable to priority groups and effective in disease control.

Finally, programme managers will recognize that under some circumstances, formal contact tracing may prejudice the establishment of a rapport between health care workers and their patients. This has occurred with some homosexual groups and in communities where the discussion of sexual contact is governed by strong negative taboos.

## Simplified contact tracing

This refers to a variety of methods by which patients identify, locate, and ensure the examination of their own sexual partners without specifically naming them to the health worker (3). Many logistic variations exist, each designed to increase the effectiveness of this system or improve its evaluation. This system overcomes some of the serious drawbacks of formal contact tracing. Simplified contact tracing actively involves the patient in the disease control effort, it is inexpensive, acceptable to patients, and reserves the limited staff time for other activities. However, the shortcomings of such patient contact referral methods include: limited effectiveness, evaluation difficulties, and low success rates with unreliable patients.

When such a system is employed, all persons who have had contact with the patient should receive the relevant information. This information should include the following:

(a) how the disease is transmitted and its incubation period,
(b) the period of infectiousness,
(c) consequences to the health of the patient and partner(s) if not treated,

(*d*) information that the sexual partner(s) needs to obtain appropriate treatment,

(*e*) the likelihood of asymptomatic infection,

(*f*) the necessity of abstaining from sex until the partner obtains a medical check-up, and

(*g*) a plan of action for each sexual partner.

The order and manner in which this information is presented will vary in each particular case, but will depend on sound educational principles (Chapter 5) (*4*).

## 8.3 Role of contact tracing

*Individual case management*

In situations where priority is placed on individual case management, some form of contact tracing has a definite role. A component of proper case management is the prevention of reinfections resulting from sexual intercourse with a partner who had not been identified and treated at the time of the first infection. Contact tracing ensures the treatment of such partners and therefore it is an essential component of individual case management.

*Control activities*

Each programme manager must balance the costs and benefits of contact tracing before adopting this control method for the entire programme. Under most circumstances some form of simplified contact tracing can be proposed because it can result in the treatment of a significant number of infected individuals at little cost. Only if a high proportion of these "contacts" were not infected would this method be excessively costly to the programme without providing disease control benefits.

Since formal contact tracing is more expensive, this activity can only be justified if the located cases are worth the cost of this activity and there are no cheaper means available.

For these reasons formal contact tracing should probably be restricted to cases having particular importance or to areas where disease prevalence is low. Special situations or groups where this more costly strategy may be worth while include: the introduction of a serious disease (e.g., syphilis or infection with penicillinase-producing *Neisseria gonorrhoeae*) into a community which was previously unaffected; all penicillinase-producing *N. gonorrhoeae* infections where control of this disease remains feasible; gonococcal pelvic inflammatory disease where a large proportion of the infected male partners are free of symptoms (*5*); females and males with repeated infections; female contacts of cases of infectious syphilis; and infections of children.

## 8.4 Selection and training of interviewers

Selection and training of interviewers will have an important influence on the effectiveness of contact tracing. The personal attributes an interviewer should possess include: an empathetic personality, the ability to communicate with people, and emotional maturity. No prior experience in the health care professions or social work is required. Such backgrounds may be valuable, but when specific skills are required, new recruits may be preferred to than those who would need retraining. Training is provided in three principal areas during in-service training courses and in handouts including information on sexually transmitted diseases, administrative procedures, and human interaction skills.

## 8.5 International contact tracing

Apart from issues of effectiveness, international (or, in federal countries, interstate) contact tracing poses an awkward situation if one programme feels compelled to respond to the needs of another programme, despite major differences in priorities.

Many countries do not even have the resources to trace local contacts, much less investigate foreign information which may be outdated, inaccurate, or irrelevant. Some proponents of this system have clearly not considered the need for the cooperation and agreement of participants prior to embarking on a costly programme which may have dubious impact and create needless ill-will between programmes. This system should be restricted to consenting participants and should preferably be mutually developed.

## 8.6 Evaluation

The evaluation of contact tracing activities has not resolved the uncertainties about its general value. Barriers to the evaluation efforts include:

(1) Widely used criteria of contact tracing effectiveness measure neither process nor outcome, and they are subject to considerable manipulation. For example "contacts elicited per interview" is not an accurate index of the appropriate process measure of elicited contacts versus actual contacts.

(2) In practice, it is extremely difficult to separate the role of contact tracing from that of many other activities. Thus, outcome measures are very difficult to obtain except in selected situations where the objectives are appropriately limited in scope.

(3) Advantages and disadvantages may be impossible to compare. For instance, it is uncertain how to compare the possible alienation of a homosexual or other high-priority person with the benefits derived from eradicating a new outbreak of syphilis or infection with penicillinase-producing *Neisseria gonorrhoeae* (PPNG).

Cost-benefit analyses are particularly difficult to use to assess the value of contact tracing. When a disease is common, the cost of detecting an individual case may be low. If a given strategy is successful and disease prevalence decreases, the cost of detecting each case may increase. Hence when a disease problem becomes minimal or when a disease is first introduced into a previously unaffected community (where contact tracing is indicated and most valuable), the cost of detecting an individual case may be enormous.

A cost-effectiveness approach overcomes some of these problems, since the actual benefit need not be estimated (Chapter 15), rather the costs of achieving a desired outcome by two different strategies are compared. This type of evaluation is essential in pilot projects before resources are committed on a larger scale.

## References

1. HEALTH EDUCATION COUNCIL. *Handbook on contact tracing in sexually transmitted diseases.* London, The Health Education Council, 1980.
2. PARRA, W. C. ET AL. Patient counselling. In: Holmes, K. K. et al., ed. *Sexually transmitted disease.* New York, McGraw Hill, 1984.
3. POTTERAT, J. J. & ROTHENBERG, R. B. The case finding effectiveness of a self-referral system for gonorrhoea: A preliminary report. *American journal of public health,* **67**: 174–176 (1977).
4. BRAMMER, L. M. & SHOSTROM, E. L. *Therapeutic psychology.* Englewood Cliffs, NJ, Prentice-Hall Inc., 1977.
5. POTTERAT, J. J. & KING, R. D. A new approach to gonorrhoea control. The asymptomatic man and incidence reduction. *Journal of the American Medical Association,* **245**: 578–580 (1981).

# Chapter 9. Clinical services

## 9.1 Introduction

Adequate management of patients and their contacts is the chief component of the control of sexually transmitted disease. However, clinical services vary widely in different settings and are often unable to provide appropriate care for patients. It is helpful to examine the use of resources (material, personnel, etc.) by the clinical services, accessibility of the services, and the population coverage of these services. However, all programmes can improve the patient care process, including patient evaluation, diagnosis, and management. The resulting improvements in the quality of the care will enhance the efficiency of the clinical services.

Some of the most common difficulties encountered in patient care are: (a) the disease conditions may not be recognized because health providers are not aware of their existence; (b) even when recognized, the problems associated with disease may not be adequately evaluated and diagnosed; (c) treatments used are often ineffective; (d) efforts to decrease the patient's risk of reinfection are inadequate or non-existent; and (e) evaluation and early treatment of sexual partners is frequently not ensured or even considered.

This chapter discusses the formal clinical services that are a part of the health system. These services are more amenable to intervention or control by public health officers or programme managers. In many countries the majority of patient care services are provided by personnel outside the established medical care system. The principles reviewed in this chapter could also be adapted and applied to these settings.

## 9.2 Principles of management

Whether patient care is provided by experts at special clinics for sexually transmitted diseases with sophisticated laboratory and technical support (e.g., as in the United Kingdom) or by primary care workers with only limited or no access to laboratory facilities (1) (e.g., many developing countries or private practitioners in some developed countries), the objectives of clinical management are the same: (a) to determine the specific cause, or the most likely etiology, of the patient's complaint or reason for attendance; (b) to provide prompt and appropriate treatment for that condition; (c) to detect other infections; (d) to ensure follow-up of the patient after treatment to determine if he or she has been cured; (e) to manage properly those patients whose treatment failed; (f) to educate the patient regarding the nature of the problem and how to avoid reinfection, and advise them to return if symptoms recur; and (*g*) to encourage the attendance of identifiable sexual partners for appropriate evaluation and treatment.

## 9.3 Practical approaches to management

Adequate care will mean that the four available strategies for control, i.e., health promotion (Chapter 5), disease detection (Chapter 6), treatment (Chapter 7), and contact tracing and patient counselling (Chapter 8), will be used to varying degrees in most cases. The availability of proper support services (Chapters 11, 12, and 13), will enhance the effectiveness, adequacy, and quality of care provided. In addition, the information from patient care activities will improve the operation of these support services, thereby contributing to overall disease control.

### Clinical setting

Even if new resources are not available to build, remodel, equip, and staff clinical facilities, improvements made to the existing clinics may still be possible. For example, a patient-flow analysis may result in the more efficient use of existing resources (*2*). Thus, a redistribution of room-use may provide increased privacy for patients during interviews and examinations; working hours can be changed to improve services for employed patients during the evening or early morning hours; assignment of specific tasks and clear responsibilities to existing personnel may increase their efficiency and decrease staff friction; etc.

### The process of care

Patients present to clinical services with clinical problems, not diagnoses. The effectiveness with which the patients' problems are resolved and disease prevention objectives are met will largely depend on the health provider's clinical acumen (this is a function of training, judgement, and experience), interpersonal skills, and the availability of support services. The provider's concern is to diagnose the patient's condition, and to decide upon the necessary management, which includes treatment type, follow-up, counselling, and outreach efforts. The use of clinical algorithms or patient management protocols may be a practical way of providing assistance to the clinicians (*3, 4*) (Annexes 2–4). Protocols can be most useful when based on a syndrome, e.g., urethritis, vaginitis, genital ulcers. However, protocols can also refer to etiological diagnoses, e.g., gonococcal urethritis, for those settings with extensive diagnostic facilities. These protocols provide a basis for clarifying personnel roles, for specifying the clinical skills required, and for planning the supplies, supervision, and other support needed by the clinical services.

*The outcome of patient care*

The process of patient care should be concerned with the resulting health status of the patient. However, depending on who is assessing the outcome of patient care, the "results" may be seen differently: (*a*) for the patient, the major concern is the alleviation of symptoms or resolution of his/her problem; (*b*) for the health provider or clinician, an acceptable outcome may be the correct diagnosis and treatment of a given patient; (*c*) for the clinic administrator, the outcome may be an efficient encounter (in terms of time and cost); (*d*) from the point of view of disease control, however, the outcome will include not only the above concerns, but also the public health aspects of disease transmission and the prevention of complications and sequelae for the individual and the community. In other words, the programme manager will wish to ensure that individual diagnosis and treatment, patient counselling, and contact tracing were all carried out.

## 9.4 Documentation

The importance of collecting information relating to the process and results of patient care cannot be overemphasized. Information gathering may be based on a standardized patient record linked to a sophisticated computer-assisted system (*5*), it may be based on a simple daily tally of patients and their problems, or it may be a daily log recording patients seen and their problems. The simplified data collection methods may include such aggregate data as the number of "males with genital ulcer" or "women with vaginal discharge" seen and treated. Whatever the level of complexity, documentation is essential to ensure effective planning for clinical services, continued quality performance, and the tracking of disease trends and epidemiology.

## 9.5 Evaluation

The evaluation of clinical services for sexually transmitted disease may focus on the structure of the service (by tabulating facilities, personnel and their qualifications, and other resources), the process of care (by record audit and direct observation), or the outcome of the service (generally by record audit). Thus, evaluations of clinical services may be characterized as quality assessment and quality assurance (*6*).

## 9.6 Principles for protocol development

As stated above, one approach to improve clinician or health provider performance is to develop and promote the widespread use of patient care algorithms for sexually transmitted disease care.

Initial efforts to develop protocols for patient care should focus on the most common problems, especially those for which diagnostic criteria and treatment are standardized. The success of efforts involving the treatment of patients by nonspecialists will largely depend on the relevance of available protocols to their daily work. Thus, the protocols should concentrate on common problems where there is enough information to provide a sound basis for the measures outlined. If there are insufficient data, priority should be given to obtaining the necessary background information.

Protocols, like treatment recommendations (Chapter 7), should always be simple and appropriate to the clinicians who will be using them. Thus, protocols requiring diagnostic tests prior to treatment should only be used by providers who have access to and actually use such tests. Similarly, protocols requiring sophisticated clinical expertise should only be formulated for those possessing these skills. For example, the ability to identify pelvic masses, a useful decision-making point in the care of women with lower abdominal pain, should only be used in protocols for those providers who possess bimanual examination skills. Likewise, the medications, referrals and contact tracing methods suggested in protocols must be relevant to the providers and setting in which they will be used.

All patient care protocols and their implementation must be periodically but regularly evaluated. The effectiveness of a protocol in influencing treatment can be inferred from its frequency of use. Infrequent use implies either that a protocol is unknown or that it is not very useful. A changing disease epidemiology and/or the cost or availability of medications, diagnostic tests, and referral opportunities all may radically alter the value of specific suggestions made in a protocol. Therefore, the protocols need to be periodically updated.

*The working group: the development of protocols*

Patient care protocols may be developed and implemented in many different ways. A multidisciplinary group is one appropriate forum for the development of protocols and the guidelines for their implementation.

This group would have a variety of tasks. First, it must assemble and analyse data on existing health care practices, the most common clinical problems associated with sexually transmitted diseases, and the providers who care for patients. Next it will be necessary to identify the evaluation techniques and diagnostic tests used by these providers. Finally, the group must understand the treatment, counselling, contact tracing, and referral practices of providers.

With this background information the group can define the problems in patient care and clarify the clinical focus for protocols and their intended users. Technical information on disease etiology, treatment efficacy, etc., and practical information (e.g., protocols developed and used in other settings) should be sought. Group consensus on protocol design is very likely to result in useful, effective, and appropriate strategies when careful attention is paid to the selection of the group members and the collection of background information.

*Implementation of patient care protocols*

The working group must also share responsibility for guiding protocol implementation. Implementation includes: provision for training or retraining health care providers; ensuring the availability of the necessary resources; evaluating protocol utility; and modifying protocols on the basis of their evaluation.

While the development of protocols is a difficult process, their adoption from other settings is usually unwise. First, the technical utility of any protocol depends on its implementation within a particular health care system to manage a specific problem. Unless the health care system and the disease epidemiology of the two settings are very similar, the "borrowed" protocol is likely to be inappropriate. Furthermore, the degree to which decision-makers support the implementation of any procedural change is directly related to their degree of involvement in developing the new policy. Hence, adoption of a protocol from elsewhere usually results in reduced commitment to its implementation.

*Evaluation of patient care protocols*

A good protocol is one that is used and guides the health provider through the process of patient management. However, the ultimate evaluation lies in the resulting health status of the patient. Examples of protocols developed for particular settings are included in Annexes 2–4.

## References

1. WHO Technical Report Series, No. 660, 1981 (*Nongonococcal urethritis and other selected sexually transmitted diseases of public health importance*: report of a WHO Scientific Group).
2. GRAVES, J. L. ET AL. Computerized patient flow analysis of local family planning clinics. *Family planning perspectives*, **13**: 164–170 (1981).
3. CHRISTENSEN-SZALANSKI, J. J. J., ET AL. Phased trial of a proven algorithm at a new primary care clinic. *American journal of public health*, **72**: 16–21 (1982).
4. MEHEUS, A. Z. Practical approaches in developing countries. In: Holmes, K. K. et al., ed. *Sexually transmitted diseases.* New York, McGraw-Hill, 1984.
5. MARGOLIS S. ET AL. Automated data entry and retrieval for health-care management. *Sexually transmitted diseases*, **8**: 211–217 (1981).
6. VUORI, H. V. *Quality assurance of health services. Concepts and methodology.* Copenhagen, World Health Organization Regional Office for Europe, 1982.

# PART III

# SUPPORT COMPONENTS

As the focus of a control programme becomes increasingly concentrated on the principal health issues related to sexually transmitted diseases and identifies priority groups, the most appropriate intervention strategies will be more clearly delineated. Likewise, as experience with these interventions develops and their direction becomes more apparent, the specific roles of the various support components will become clearer. In addition, as support components evolve they can indicate new approaches for existing interventions, making them even more effective.

Thus, a prevention centre for sexually transmitted diseases (Chapter 10) provides the multidisciplinary expertise necessary for an effective programme. Furthermore, as a focus for the development and testing of new disease detection methods and patient management protocols, this component can directly contribute to control programme plans.

Similarly, a well-developed information system (Chapter 11) will enhance the programme by documenting disease and activity trends efficiently and accurately. The innovative use of available information will clarify the principal health issues of the diseases and will aid in the identification of priority groups. Since these health issues and priority groups undergo revision, rapid use of data may be crucial to programme efficiency and effectiveness.

Professional training (Chapter 12) or the training of health workers is an important aspect in developing personnel skills for control activities. As training expertise improves and programme expectations increase, the skills that are vital to control will be more clearly delineated for a variety of health workers. The training process is a cooperative effort of programme managers and trainers who together identify programme performance problems and clarify those that are due to a lack of skills.

The laboratory system (Chapter 13) is important for surveillance activities, the development of treatment recommendations and patient management protocols, disease detection efforts, and often the diagnosis of individual cases. As this system improves, new opportunities for disease intervention will develop. Thus, testing antenatal patients for syphilis can only be undertaken as an intervention when serological testing becomes generally available.

# Chapter 10. Centres for prevention of sexually transmitted diseases

## 10.1 Introduction

Effective control programmes coordinate many different disciplines and activities. A disease prevention centre has an important place in the integration of numerous functions: improving clinical care, improving laboratory diagnosis, developing programmes for the training of health care personnel, and performing relevant operational research.

The prevention centre should be the central point for all activities relating to sexually transmitted diseases. Its size and geographical localization are not important. The expertise needed for the centre to function effectively includes a mixture of clinical, epidemiological, laboratory, and social science skills, although none of these are an absolute requirement. Local exigencies will dictate the mixture of expertise required.

## 10.2 Functions of the centre

*Improving clinical care.*

The prevention centre should assist in the effort to ensure that clinical care for patients with sexually transmitted diseases is effective. This may involve widely different settings for health care delivery, ranging from the primary care level to special clinics, and different specific national priorities for control. In all of these activities, the prevention centre should involve potential users in the development of activities and should test protocols prior to their official acceptance. The following are the tasks the centre will have to carry out:

(1) *Identify the providers of care and determine their practices.* This profile of practices and providers can be detailed to completely describe the setting as was done in Seattle (*1, 2*). In other situations, a survey can focus on "special clinics", particularly when most care is provided in such facilities (*3, 4*). Less formal approaches may be more appropriate in developing nations and could include infirmary reviews, discussions with key villagers, and selected patient surveys.

(2) *Develop protocols for the clinical evaluation and follow-up of patients.* Protocols should be developed which encompass history taking, physical examination, taking of specimens, and interpreting and recording results. These protocols should be based on the common disease presentations. Several different versions may be necessary for care providers with different training, skills, and resources.

(3) *Make public the treatment recommendations for the sexually transmitted diseases of major concern.* Though some nations have developed treatment guidelines for these diseases none may be appropriate *per se* in other countries (Chapter 7). Treatment will be determined by the resources available and logistic considerations, and by the cultural features and specific epidemiological circumstances of the country. The centre can greatly assist in guideline development, with operational research, and in the promulgation of guidelines once developed, through its training and standard-setting roles.

(4) *Determine appropriate approaches to patient counselling and contact tracing for the clinical care system* (see Chapter 8). A wide choice of methods are available for counselling and contact tracing procedures. Methods must be tailored to the specific circumstances. In industrialized nations, a complex computer-based system may be feasible for patient tracking. In some nations, individual patient follow-up may not be possible on any level.

## Improving laboratory diagnostic support

In conjunction with the laboratory service system the prevention centre can set the diagnostic standards and specify the laboratory needs for patient care. The centre can also provide the necessary support for the laboratory system. This will involve:

(1) *Identifying the laboratory tests that should be routinely available for patient care.* Patient care protocols will specify laboratory tests for the various problems at each particular level of care. The parallel development of clinical skills and laboratory tests will ensure that the protocols are useful.

(2) *Assisting in the development of appropriate diagnostic tests where none exist at present.* The rapid plasma-reagin card test (RPR) was developed as a syphilis screening test that is rapid and requires minimal laboratory sophistication, a need which was identified by control programmes (see Annex 1). Likewise, selective media were needed to culture the organisms causing gonorrhoea in order to further gonorrhoea control efforts (6). The centre facilitates laboratory development by specifying needs and by providing operational research opportunities.

(3) *Cooperating with the laboratory system to assess resource needs, document test procedures, and develop continuous evaluation methods for diagnostic tests.* A system will also be needed so that problematical diagnostic specimens can be referred.

## Developing training programmes

The role of the centre in establishing standards for clinical and laboratory services is intimately linked to its training function. Appropriate patient care protocols are a basis for specifying the responsibilities of various health workers. Such an analysis leads directly to the objectives for training these personnel and for evaluating their performance after training. Similarly, training for laboratory personnel can be based on the specified routine tests to be performed. The training efforts of the centre should include provision for health workers at all levels.

In addition to these training functions, the prevention centre should assume responsibility for disseminating information to all who are interested in sexually transmitted diseases. The topics covered should include updates on disease trends, epidemiology, diagnostic procedures, treatment recommendations, contact tracing, and effective methods of patient education. Since this information is intended for a variety of audiences, several different formats will be necessary. Press releases, for example, reach a broad spectrum of individuals and may greatly assist in mobilizing public support for disease control efforts. Publications of all kinds including medical and paramedical journals, ministry of health reports, surveillance reports, and other special publications for health workers should be used to inform colleagues. Presentations to various lay and health-worker groups will also assist in highlighting topics related to sexually transmitted diseases and the plans for control.

## Developing operational research

Finally, the centre is in an ideal position to identify, conduct, and analyse special studies needed to support the control programme. Its multidisciplinary structure (with epidemiological, clinical, and laboratory expertise) is geared to assessing the multiple aspects of control given below:

(1) *Clinical studies.* The centre should design operational research studies to evaluate diagnostic procedures and treatment recommendations. These studies begin with the assessment of current diagnostic and treatment practices used by most care providers. Subsequent studies can evaluate these practices and modifications to obtain feasible, acceptable standards. Intervention strategies must be studied in order to ensure that they are appropriate and effective (7). Surveillance of trends in gonococcal susceptibilities (8) and prevalence of penicillinase-producing gonococci (9) can easily be conducted at existing clinics. Of equal importance are studies designed to identify the methods that are effective in obtaining the referral of sexual partners and which help patients to adopt preventive health behaviour (10).

(2) *Epidemiological studies.* For epidemiological studies, an accurate assessment of the incidence of sexually transmitted disease can be based upon a selected sample of facilities with diagnostic and data collection capabilities. Particular emphasis should be placed on studying disease problems at the primary health care level. Point-prevalence studies of selected groups (e.g., pregnant women, prostitutes, military personnel, and students) for infection or seroreactivity may be useful. Case-control or cohort studies may provide more useful information and should be introduced if resources and expertise permit. Studies to evaluate the impact of pilot control efforts will be required.

*Managing specialized clinics*

A clinic for sexually transmitted diseases, sponsored and managed by the prevention centre, may enhance many of the centre's functions. Direct patient care experience will facilitate protocol development (*11*) and small-scale evaluations prior to field testing. Laboratory development will be aided by direct experience with a clinic laboratory, which would provide correlations between clinical and laboratory data. These laboratory and clinical resources may support some operational and epidemiological research needs of the control programme. Training activities will also benefit from the existence of a special clinic. The assistance of experienced clinic personnel will be invaluable for the trainers when preparing curricula and programmes for health personnel.

A cautionary note—a clinic can be an asset to the overall efforts of the prevention centre, but may pose two problems: (1) the patient population in a specialized clinic may not be representative of the total population; (2) the clinic tends to absorb resources and may become the central focus of the control activities, to the exclusion of other functions and other geographical areas. Planners must guard against the isolation and elitism that can result when there is a single central clinic. The prevention centre is a mixture of elements, with no absolute requirements, but with a mandate to consider the overall problem.

## References

1. GALE, J. L. & HINDS, M. W. Male urethritis in King County, Washington, 1974–75: I. Incidence. *American journal of public health*, **68**: 20–25 (1978).
2. HINDS, M. W. & GALE, J. L. Male urethritis in King County, Washington, 1974–75: II. Diagnosis and treatment. *American journal of public health*, **68**: 26–30 (1978).
3. ADLER, M. W. & Diagnostic, treatment and reporting criteria for non-specific genital infection in sexually transmitted disease clinics in England and Wales 1: Diagnosis. *British journal of venereal diseases*, **54**: 422–427 (1978).
4. BELSEY, E. M. & ADLER, M. W. Study of STD clinic attenders in England and Wales, 1978: 2 Patterns of diagnosis. *British journal of venereal diseases*, **57**: 290–294 (1981).
5. PORTNOY, J. Modifications of the Rapid Plasma Reagin (RPR) Card test for syphilis, for use in large scale testing. *American journal of clinical pathology*, **40**: 473–479 (1963).
6. THAYER, J. D. & MARTIN Jr., J. E. Improved medium selective for cultivation of *N. gonorrhoeae* and *N. meningitidis*. *Public health reports*, **81**: 559–562 (1966).
7. MEHEUS, A. Z. Practical approaches in developing countries. In: Holmes, K. K. et al., ed. *Sexually transmitted diseases*. New York, McGraw-Hill, 1984.
8. GUINAN, M. E. ET AL. The national gonorrhoea therapy monitoring study: I. Review of treatment results and in-vitro antibiotic susceptibility, 1972–1978. *Sexually transmitted diseases*, **6**: 93–102 (1979).
9. BROWN, S. T. ET AL. Antimicrobial resistance of *Neisseria gonorrhoeae* in Bangkok: Is single drug treatment passé? *Lancet*, **2**: 1366–1368 (1982).
10. PARRA, W. C., ET AL. Patient counselling. In: Holmes, K. K. et al., ed. *Sexually transmitted diseases*. New York, McGraw-Hill, 1984.
11. CENTERS FOR DISEASE CONTROL. *Guidelines for a quality assurance system in community-sponsored sexually transmitted diseases clinics*. Atlanta, Department of Health and Human Services, CDC, 1981 (No. 00–3878).

# Chapter 11. Information systems

## 11.1 Introduction

The term "information system" encompasses everything from high speed communications and electronic data processing to oral tradition. However, some type of system at whatever level is a prerequisite for effective programme planning, coordination, budgeting, monitoring, and evaluation. The choice of an information system depends on the resources, and the costs and programme benefits of the alternatives. The "correct" choice is the one that uses a technology appropriate to local circumstances.

## 11.2 Types of system

The first objective of a data system is to define the size of the problem and its distribution in time, place, and person. Three types of data system can interact for this purpose: clinician notification, laboratory notification, and sentinel and *ad hoc* surveillance. The second important task is a management-oriented information system (MIS) that focuses on the process of control rather than the epidemiology of disease. This system attempts to answer three questions: (*a*) What is being done? (*b*) Does it have the desired effect? (*c*) What happens when it is changed?

The following sections discuss briefly the nature and purpose of information systems for sexually transmitted diseases. Design features are not included, not only because of their overwhelming detail, but to stress the importance of local resources and logistics in finding appropriate solutions.

## 11.3 Systems for epidemiology

*Clinician notification*

A variety of clinicians see patients suffering from sexually transmitted diseases (specialists in venereology, other specialists, general practitioners, non-physician clinicians, etc.), and are therefore potential reporters of disease cases. The precision and detail of the notification is a function of the interest and sophistication of the clinician. On all levels, however, regular notification will occur only if the system is simple and provides for periodic feedback to the clinicians.

When developing a notification system for the programme, managers must identify: the providers; the data which are feasible for them to provide; the transmittal method; the data users; and feedback systems to the provider. Simplified notification systems have been proposed for and used by providers in areas without access to diagnostic tests (2, 3). These suggest that notifications can be subdivided by sex (male, female), by large age-groups (under 15, 15–29, 30 years and over) and by syndrome (urethral discharge, vaginal discharge, genital ulcer). In contrast, in the United Kingdom, clinics report a wide variety of specific diagnostic categories by sex and by 5-year age-groups (4). Obviously the latter notification system provides more precise epidemiological detail but requires sophisticated clinical and laboratory services and substantial data collection resources.

At these extremes, the notification system has been developed to meet the needs of a particular setting. The simplified system used in Swaziland allows calculation of the occurrence of sexually transmitted disease in a population, and projection of the medication supplies required for health units (5). The detailed information available in the United Kingdom allows the venereologist to measure disease trends more precisely. In both settings these data are also used as the basis of public information exercises. Thus, the simplified system is just as useful for assessing disease trends and providing management information in those areas where it is the appropriate system to be used. The quality of a system does not depend on the technology used but is related to the thoroughness with which the required data are obtained, the accessibility of the data, and the usefulness of the information to programme managers.

In any system, some attention must be paid to certain epidemiological problems. For example, some workers have emphasized the importance of separating the number of disease cases from the number of patients with sexually transmitted disease (6). Patients may have several concurrent infections, multiple episodes of one or more diseases within a given time period, or may have a relapsing infection. This over-representation of individuals may obscure both the actual situation with regard to the correct epidemiology of the diseases and the target groups involved in disease transmission. Computerized data systems with unique patient identifiers and record linkage may solve some of these problems (7), but a well-designed manual system can also avoid some of the epidemiological distortion.

Another important pitfall is the misclassification of sexual partners who receive treatment without diagnosis. Counting these individuals as either cases or as having "other conditions requiring treatment" obscures important aspects of disease control (4). The common denominator for these, and a variety of other epidemiological mishaps, is a failure to obtain a consensus on case definition and reporting convention at the outset and a failure to reconsider these aspects periodically.

*Laboratory notification*

Though laboratory confirmation of cases is ideal, a separate, parallel laboratory and clinical notification system can result in duplication and may require the linking of records to avoid this problem. Either the clinician or the laboratory staff, preferably the former, should assume responsibility for the official notification system.

On the other hand, the laboratory may provide important adjuncts to official reporting. The number of positive isolates, positive serological tests, and specimens processed is a useful indicator of overall activity and a cross-check on official notification. If more sophisticated data processing is available, a one-to-one correlation may be undertaken (e.g., syphilis registries in the USA) between laboratory reports and official notification. Laboratory reporting has its greatest impact in the rapid identification of microbiological changes (e.g., the emergence of penicillinase-producing *Neisseria gonorrhoeae* (PPNG)) and the periodic monitoring of anti-microbial susceptibility patterns.

Finally, laboratory surveillance can be used as a check on clinical activity, through smear-culture correlation and comparisons between clinics and clinicians. Thus, the laboratory may provide a sensitive early warning system of changes in clinical practice or breaks in technique.

## Sentinel and ad hoc *surveillance*

No routine notification system identifies all cases of infection. A method for identifying the notification biases is also required in order to extrapolate the results obtained to the entire population. Sentinel surveillance systems and/or *ad hoc* surveys can be used to identify these reporting biases, supplementing the notifications received. Such methods may even be an alternative to routine reporting since, in some settings, such periodic efforts may be less costly than developing and maintaining an ongoing notification system.

(1) *Sentinel surveillance.* Sentinel surveillance is the identification of representative health care facilities that perform pre-defined disease tests on their patients and report the results to the control programme. Selection of the sentinel facilities, the tests to be done, and the reporting format will depend upon the setting. If the system is established with care it will be possible to estimate from the data the disease prevalence in the population. The advantages of such a system are that the number of providers is limited, reporting biases are minimized, and feedback of information to the providers is simplified.

Such sentinel surveillance facilities could ultimately be expanded to provide more detailed information than is feasible in traditional notification systems. Finally, these sentinel sites could be developed into a system providing useful information concerning protocol effectiveness, treatment efficacy, and antimicrobial monitoring (8).

Surveillance systems developed for other purposes may be utilized as well. For example, in the United States of America the hospital discharge summary data provide an ongoing measure of pelvic inflammatory disease in the whole country (9). Such discharge summaries may also be used to follow trends of ectopic pregnancies and other conditions.

(2) *Ad hoc surveys.* Periodic surveys may also be used to supplement other data sources. Thus, for example, periodic surveys conducted in

Swaziland enabled programme managers to identify etiological diagnoses among patients with urethral discharge, vaginal discharge, or genital ulcer disease (*3, 10*). Other *ad hoc* surveys have identified the etiology of acute pelvic inflammatory disease, clearly documenting the gonococcus as an important cause of this syndrome (*11, 12*).

Population-based sample surveys may also be used to identify the true distribution of disease in a particular setting. Such surveys are very expensive and are generally of limited use for sexually transmitted disease programmes. However, when other surveys are being conducted, the addition of related items may be feasible. Such opportunities should be used whenever possible.

## 11.4 Systems for management

Information systems useful to the control programme need to identify not only the status of disease and disease trends, but also the processes of the control programme itself. In fact, measures of the process may be more useful to programme managers than measures of the outcome. To be effective, the information system must provide timely information to correct deficiencies and reward competence.

The inputs for this system (*7*) may be as detailed as circumstances permit but should include information on activities, resource utilization, and task accomplishment of programme personnel. The outputs should be related to predefined programme goals, and the designers should attempt to produce questions for which there is a single answer (How many cases were interviewed and dispositioned? How many villages were visited? How many culture plates were contaminated? etc.). In any setting, the system should be built around a small number of questions that have to be answered. Even if data processing resources are available, the information system should be expanded with care and only when this expansion can be shown to be useful to the control effort.

## References

1. MEHEUS, A. Z. ET AL. Evaluation of notification of venereal diseases as a basis for contact tracing in Belgium. *Tijdschrift voor social geneeskunde*, **54**: 22–25 (1976).
2. ARY, O. P. ET AL. *Tropical venereology*, Edinburgh, Churchill Livingstone, 1980.
3. MEHEUS, A. Z. Practical approaches in developing nations. In: Holmes, K. K. et al., ed. *Sexually transmitted diseases*. New York, McGraw-Hill, 1984.
4. ADLER, M. W. Diagnostic, treatment and reporting criteria for gonorrhoea in sexually transmitted disease clinics in England and Wales 2: Treatment and reporting criteria. *British journal of venereal disease*, **54**: 15–23 (1978).
5. MEHEUS, A. ET AL. Genital infections in Swaziland. *Annales de la Société belge de médecine tropicale*, **62**: 361–367 (1982).
6. BELSEY, E. M. & ADLER, M. W. Study of STD clinic attenders in England and Wales, 1978: 1. Patients versus cases. *British journal of venereal diseases*, **57**: 285–289 (1981).
7. FICHTNER, R. R. ET AL. A statewide management information system for the control of sexually transmitted diseases. *Proceedings of the First STD World Congress, Puerto Rico, November 1981*.

8. WHO Technical Report Series, No. 660, 1981 (*Nongonococcal urethritis and other selected sexually transmitted diseases of public health importance*: report of a WHO Scientific Group).

9. JONES, O. G. ET AL. Frequency and distribution of salpingitis and pelvic inflammatory disease in short-stay hospitals in the United States. *American journal of obstetrics and gynecology*, **138**: 905–908 (1980).

10. MEHEUS, A. ET AL. Epidemiology and aetiology of urethritis in Swaziland. *International journal of epidemiology*, **9**: 239–245 (1980).

11. RATNAM, A. V. ET AL. Gonococcal infection in women with pelvic inflammatory disease in Lusaka, Zambia. *American journal of obstetrics and gynecology*, **138**: 965–968 (1980).

12. RENDTORFF, R. C. ET AL. Economic consequences of gonorrhoea in women: Experience from an urban hospital. *Journal of the American Venereal Disease Association*, **1**: 40–47 (1974).

# Chapter 12. Professional training

## 12.1 Introduction

Over the last two decades, the training of medical personnel in the diagnosis, treatment, and prevention of sexually transmitted diseases has not kept pace with the observed increase in the incidence of these diseases in most countries. Currently, in both industrialized and developing nations, training ranges from inadequate to non-existent (*1–3*).

The problems are complex. The spectrum of health personnel involved in disease control depends largely on the organization of the health services. Some countries have a well-established network of clinics, and the majority of patients are treated by physicians under the supervision of a trained venereologist. In other countries, general practitioners and medical specialists other than venereologists treat the majority of patients, often in their private practices. In most developing countries there is a general shortage of physicians and most cases are treated by nurses, paramedical personnel, pharmacists, and traditional healers.

Thus, the development of training must be linked to the social setting, the pre-existing system for medical care, and the established mechanisms for medical training. An incremental approach, with specific definable goals, is required for the gradual assimilation of the principles of the control of sexually transmitted disease by the medical community.

## 12.2 Academic training

*Medical school training*

Instruction in the management and control of sexually transmitted diseases should be included in any medical school curriculum. A minimum of 20 hours of training in venereology should include lectures and seminars, outpatient sessions, microbiological and serological demonstrations, discussions with contact tracers and social workers, and formal lectures in epidemiology and methods of control (*1*). The teaching should include an appreciation of the broad spectrum of human sexual relationships and as much patient contact as possible.

Case studies are useful and role-playing exercises in which the student can participate both as interviewer and as patient are valuable in providing a controlled setting for the early stages of learning (*4*). The study of these diseases can be made part of a comprehensive training in human sexuality, which should include family planning, contraception, the varieties of sexual expression, and the psychological foundation for sexual counselling.

In many parts of the world, venereology is considered a minor subject, divided among dermatologists, urologists, and gynaecologists (5). In the United Kingdom, sexually transmitted diseases are the responsibility of the venereologist, who coordinates a multidisciplinary team. In countries where this integrating role is not filled by a venereologist, the identification of and agreement on a coordinating faculty member may be difficult. This role could be assumed, for example, by the person responsible for training in general practice, community medicine, infectious diseases, or human sexuality.

## Paramedical school training

In developing countries the majority of patients are seen, evaluated, and treated by auxiliary health workers, i.e., nurses, pharmacists, medical auxiliaries, laboratory technicians, health inspectors, social workers, etc. It is crucial that theoretical and practical instruction in the paramedical institutions bear a realistic relationship to their future facilities and role.

Organized instruction should include the diagnosis and management of the diseases, epidemiology and control, and organization of services where the student will work. Auxiliary personnel should also be taught the basic principles of contact tracing and the use and operation of standing orders to assist in unsupervised patient management. The provision of concise, well-illustrated instruction manuals, algorithms, charts, slides, etc., is usually of great help. Such aids should be selected for their relevance to the cultural background of the students, as well as for their appropriateness to the course and available facilities.

## Postgraduate training

The United Kingdom is probably the only major country in the world where venereology is recognized and practiced as a separate specialty (1, 6). Consequently, the specialist training there is the best organized. The need for a recognized diploma in venereology and genitourinary medicine (1) has led to the development of two full-time, 3-month courses in the United Kingdom (in Liverpool and London) (6). Other countries have organized postgraduate courses as well. A vigorous postgraduate training programme can modify patient care practices of clinicians, including sexual partner care. The training can also result in improved notification by practising clinicians and a heightened awareness of the problem. An attempt should be made to ensure that this training reaches practising clinicians in remote areas as well as those located near the training institution. In addition, the control programme should ideally become integrated into all types of continuing education systems.

## In-service training

Although formal academic programmes are important, they cannot replace the less formal in-service refresher training that occurs at the work place. A variety of formats of this type of training are available, including the travelling seminar, local publications, exchange of personnel, radio or television programmes, etc. The training can be geared to the professional level and expertise of the audience (e.g., physician, nurse, medical assistant), and should be open to other health care workers in the area who might be involved with some aspect of sexually transmitted diseases. If feasible, it is recommended that a regular and repeated programme is planned for in-service training, to maintain interest and continuing expectations (7, 8).

In many developing countries, the key people to whom in-service training must be directed are primary health care workers and their supervisors (9–11). Since these workers may provide care for most of the nation, integration of work associated with sexually transmitted diseases into their activities becomes a prime focus for the control effort.

Finally, although this chapter has concentrated on the training of clinicians, other groups including laboratory workers (see Chapter 13), managers, field investigators, and health educators, should also be considered in overall training programmes. For each group, the development of formal educational systems and ongoing in-service training is indispensable for an effective control programme.

## 12.3 Overall strategy

To implement its training requirements, the control programme should consider the following elements:

(1) The first priority is the training of the staff of the prevention centre to form a group of competent and well-motivated individuals to undertake much of the planning and implementation of the programme. Training should focus on simple ways of measuring the magnitude of the problem, setting specific goals, and specifying the needs and plans appropriate to the country.

(2) National training activities should commence as soon as a national control programme has been formulated, the technologies to be applied at the various levels of the health service have been decided upon, and training objectives for the various categories of health personnel identified.

(3) Training should be practical and relevant to the environment in which health workers will be exercising their newly-acquired skills. Thus, national training capacities should be rapidly developed, in cooperation with regional and international resources.

(4) To promote interaction among physicians, laboratory workers, and peripheral health workers, it is crucial that group educational activities should provide the opportunity for an exchange of ideas.

(5) Students in all medical schools should receive training in a clinic for sexually transmitted diseases, with the specialist responsible for the care of patients serving as their teacher.

(6) Special emphasis should be put on teaching obstetrician gynaecologists and paediatricians to recognize sexually transmitted diseases and to be aware of their consequences for their patients.

# References

1. CATERALL, R. D. Education of physicians in the sexually transmitted diseases in the United Kingdom. *British journal of venereal diseases*, **52**: 97–99 (1976).
2. STAMM, W. E. ET AL. Clinical training in venereology in the United States and Canada. *Journal of the American Medical Association*, **248**: 2020–2024 (1982).
3. ADLER, M. & WILLCOX, R. R. Teaching of genitourinary medicine (venereology) to undergraduate medical students in Britain. *British journal of venereal diseases*, **57**: 170–173 (1981).
4. MACE, R. H. O. ET AL. *The teaching of human sexuality in schools for health professionals.* Geneva, World Health Organization, 1974 (Public Health Papers No. 57).
5. DELME, H. The role of the practitioner, public health officer, dermatologist and other specialists in the teaching, investigations and treatment of STD: the situation in the Common Market countries. *British journal of venereal diseases*, **52**: 107–109 (1976).
6. ALERGANT, C. D. A diploma in venereology. *British journal of venereal diseases*, **46**: 162–163 (1970).
7. WEBSTER, B. The medical manpower situation in the United States in relation to sexually transmitted diseases. *British journal of venereal diseases*, **52**: 94–96 (1976).
8. WILLCOX, R. R. VD education in developing countries: a comparison with developed countries. *British journal of venereal diseases*, **52**: 88–93 (1976).
9. MCMAHON, R. ET AL. *On being in charge. A guide for middle-level management in primary health care.* Geneva, World Health Organization, 1980.
10. *The primary health worker* (revised edition). Geneva, World Health Organization, 1980.
11. WERNER, D. *Where there is no doctor.* London, Macmillan Press Ltd., 1979.

# Chapter 13. Laboratory services

## 13.1 Introduction

Laboratory services are an integral part of all control programmes. While a few countries have specific laboratory support for their control programmes, most provide these services through the general laboratory system.

Laboratory services perform diagnostic tests which aid individual case management. Screening and case-finding activities usually depend on laboratory tests. Furthermore, laboratory services are an essential support for identifying the disease problem, clarifying its distribution, developing new control technologies, and monitoring disease trends.

## 13.2 Barriers

Several barriers impede the development of effective laboratory services for the control of sexually transmitted disease. The most important problem in many countries is the limited funds allocated for laboratory services and the low prestige accorded to laboratory medicine. In addition, other programmes competing for these scarce resources are often given priority. Staffing is often inadequate both in numbers and the skills required to perform the required tests. Similarly, equipment is frequently lacking or cannot be used because repairs are not carried out. Reagents are often imported, expensive, and in short supply.

Barriers are also created by poor planning. A lack of coordination between the control programme and the laboratory system hamper the effective use of those laboratory services that are available. Thus, the laboratory services available may be inappropriate to the purposes of the programme because the tests are unhelpful, results are excessively delayed, or tests are unavailable where most patient-care decisions are made. Finally, in the absence of coordinated planning, laboratory services support may not be available for those special studies that are required to define the disease problem and to develop appropriate control strategies.

## 13.3 Responsibilities

A distinction should be made between specialized laboratory services provided by the prevention centre and the routine patient care and screening services provided by the general laboratory system. The former emphasize developmental work; the latter concentrate on the laboratory

72

support needs of the care providers *vis à vis* the control of sexually transmitted diseases.

## 13.4 Programme planning

Managers of the control programme and the laboratory system must jointly review disease problems and develop programme objectives. Such a review should include an assessment of the resources available within the health system for laboratory services. First, managers need to examine their priorities so that they can determine what laboratory services can be supported within the existing budgets. When adequate funds are not available, managers must endeavour to obtain new resources.

Control strategies should be described in sufficient detail so that precise task descriptions can be produced for all levels of health care providers. The plan must make clear which routine diagnostic services will be available for control purposes at which facilities. This joint planning must include provision for cases where management is based on clinical or epidemiological assessment and does not depend upon the use of diagnostic tests. In these situations, the success or failure of such schemes must be periodically assessed. These evaluations will provide both data and an opportunity to review whether the scheme should be continued or whether diagnostic tests should now be made available.

## 13.5 Implementation

The manager of the laboratory system will be responsible for implementing the diagnostic tests that have been agreed upon. Precise descriptions of the test procedures, including quality control methods, must be recorded and laboratory personnel responsible for performing or supervising the tests should, therefore be trained in record-keeping.

As resources become available, the manager must plan for the incorporation of new tests into the system. Using the procedure descriptions, managers can derive a specific task description for each laboratory worker, and incorporate appropriate training of personnel in the necessary skills. Supervisory personnel must also become familiar with the new tests, the quality assessment measures to be used, and effective training methods for the new skills. The control programme manager and the laboratory system manager must coordinate the implementation of new procedures to ensure that health care providers obtain specimens correctly, transmit them properly to the laboratory, and interpret the laboratory test results correctly.

The manager of the laboratory system is responsible for integrating the various parts of the system. This integration seeks to unify the various levels of laboratory services, reflecting the different capabilities and responsibilities of each part. The aim is to obtain maximum efficiency and effectiveness of the overall laboratory services. Effective two-way communication is essential for the efficient operation of this system.

*Peripheral laboratories*

Peripheral laboratories (defined functionally) are those having limited capabilities. Each is usually staffed by one person, who may be trained to perform a limited number of functions, e.g., peripheral blood counts and smear examinations. Such laboratories may be found in sexually transmitted disease clinics, private practitioners' offices, or outpatient services. Equipment is limited, usually restricted to a bright-field microscope and appropriate supplies. Dark-field microscopy is desirable in settings where genital ulcers commonly occur.

*Intermediate laboratories*

Laboratories at this level have increased capabilities, including the ability to culture and perform some serological tests. The work at such laboratories is performed by a team of workers, frequently handling problems referred from smaller laboratories. In general, they will also have some supervisory relationship with the smaller laboratories. With greater resources, these laboratories are considerably more versatile than the peripheral ones. Many of the investigations at this level are assisted by hospital laboratories.

*Central laboratories*

These are generally well equipped and the staff highly skilled. Such laboratories usually serve as national research and reference centres. Many university research laboratories function at this level of competence. Due to prohibitive costs, certain investigations which are potentially available at these facilities cannot be performed frequently. The use of such expensive tests should be carefully planned, including selection of patients and problems to be studied, and the numbers limited to what is necessary to answer specific questions. Many such investigations will be research-oriented.

A national central laboratory has several other important functions apart from diagnosis and research. These include training laboratory personnel, operating quality control programmes, and ensuring smooth functioning and coordination of the entire laboratory system. The central laboratory must carefully assess its available manpower and resources. Some may find it more efficient to delegate the more complex technical investigations to university research laboratories, while retaining the training quality control and supervisory functions.

*Quality control*

To ensure uniform, high quality laboratory services, procedures must be standardized and all reagents tested against controls first. Control sera should be used to check on serological procedures.

## 13.6 Evaluation and quality assurance

The laboratory system manager will often have developed a quality assurance procedure for its general programme of work. The laboratory services provided must be included in this general quality assurance system. Attention must be given to delays in reporting test results, test utilization, and resource wastage. It should be used to identify performance problems and their cause and should indicate specific ways of resolving these problems. A quality assurance programme is a necessity even for a laboratory system with very limited resources.

The control programme and the laboratory system must be closely coordinated. Observed changes in disease problems and priorities will ultimately result in alterations in the control strategies and may require different laboratory diagnostic services. Such changes will result from evaluations which indicate barriers to programme effectiveness that were not initially appreciated. In addition, new disease patterns, treatment problems, and new diagnostic techniques will undoubtedly occur and will require new approaches to laboratory services.

## 13.7 A pragmatic approach

The guiding principle for laboratory services must be that they enhance the control and effectiveness of the programme for sexually transmitted diseases. The least expensive methods capable of achieving this end should be selected. For example, periodic field surveys may be cheaper and more feasible than establishing the performance of routine diagnostic tests where they do exist at present. Where a variety of alternative tests exist, the cost and benefits of each must be considered before a particular one is selected. In general, as tests become more sensitive and specific, they also become

**Table 5.** Laboratory test performance at various levels of the laboratory system

| Etiological agent | Laboratory test[a] | Level | | |
|---|---|---|---|---|
| | | peripheral | intermediate | central |
| *Neisseria gonorrhoeae* | Gram-stain smear | + | + | + |
| | Culture isolation | | + | + |
| | β-lactamase testing | | +/− | + |
| | Susceptibility testing | | | + |
| | Typing | | | +/− |
| *Treponema pallidum* | Dark-field microscopy | +/− | + | + |
| | RPR card test (qualitative) | +/− | + | + |
| | VDRL (quantitative) | | + | + |
| | TPHA (qualitative) | | | + |
| | Other: FTA-ABS, TPI | | | +/− |

[a] RPR card test = rapid plasma-reagin card test.
VDRL = Venereal Disease Research Laboratory.
TPHA = *Treponema pallidum* haemagglutination assay.
FTA-ABS = Fluorescent treponemal antibody absorbed test.
TPI = *Treponema pallidum* immobilization test.

more complex and require more expensive material and greater technological expertise. The least expensive and simplest test capable of providing the required information should be selected.

The laboratory system must support the objectives of the control programme. If, for example, control priorities target highly specific problems, then laboratory support services should match these. Nevertheless, there will always be a need for research work which will ultimately lead to new control priorities. Laboratory activities at the various service levels outlined above need to be integrated. An example of an integrated laboratory scheme for two common sexually transmitted diseases is shown in Table 5.

# PART IV

# IMPLEMENTATION

The aim of the control programme for sexually transmitted diseases is the prevention of ill-health resulting from these conditions through various interventions. These interventions may have a primary prevention focus (the prevention of infection), a secondary prevention focus (minimizing the adverse health effects of infection), or usually a combination of the two. While tertiary prevention is also important in limiting the effects of disabilities caused by disease, it has little relevance to the control of sexually transmitted diseases.

Effective disease control requires the interaction of a large number of people performing different tasks in a particular time sequence. To organize these efforts, ensuring that the required personnel, personnel skills, and material resources are available, requires careful programme management. Although the technical details of control are different from those of other health programmes, the management skills are often quite similar. Whenever possible, disease control programmes should attempt to apply management approaches which have proved to be successful within the particular local setting.

A crucial aspect of effective management is the monitoring of disease trends and programme activities. Evaluation will show if the activities have been performed in an accurate, prompt and satisfactory way. The information obtained will identify performance problems and can be used to make the necessary changes required to improve control efforts. Ongoing evaluation of disease trends provides a more direct measure of programme effectiveness and may be used to determine the appropriateness of the selected intervention strategies for a particular setting.

# Chapter 14. Programme management

## 14.1 Introduction

Programme management ensures that the objectives of the programme are achieved. The first steps in initiating either a new programme or revised directions in an existing programme will be to establish control priorities reflecting the disease problems, technical feasibility of control, available resources, and the commitment of the government and community. The process of describing priorities will lead to a consideration of the control strategies available and result in the selection of a particular strategy or a combination of several strategies.

The next step in developing the new or revised control programme will be to plan the intervention activities. Since control strategies usually involve a large number of people and groups, such plans may be quite complex and will reflect the need for long-term coordinated development. Many required activities will depend on individuals whose principal duties and responsibilities are not directly involved in the control programme. These new actions should, therefore, be negotiated in advance to ensure their effective integration into the overall programme effort.

One approach to developing implementation plans is to describe an overall work system. Such a system begins with an analysis of the tasks which must be performed to ensure that the strategies are achieved. On the basis of this task analysis, it will be possible to describe the resources required and the system necessary for managing these resources. This overall system will define job descriptions for each individual and this will ensure that adequate resources and people are available, and that staff are trained and supervised in the activities needed.

Developing the plan for a workable, comprehensive management system may be difficult and time-consuming. However, the completed plan can assist in the discussions with others so that roles and expectations can be clarified, negotiated, and restructured. The complexities of this task can be diminished by focusing on the more modest first-year goals which may concentrate on a pilot or demonstration activity or an activity which has a limited geographical or technical focus. Inevitably the initial experience will provide a more realistic basis for the planning of future extensions of the control programme.

## 14.2 Design strategies

On the basis of the intervention(s) selected, detailed plans for the first years activities can be made together with a general description of long-term plans. The place(s) where these activities will be conducted must be specified. The population and disease problems at that site can then be estimated. Using these estimates, the resources required for the interventions can be calculated and the proportion already available can be projected. A feasible date can then be selected for the intervention to begin.

The programme targets selected should be both realistic and reflect a level of performance that will result in health improvement. Process targets which reflect population coverage, performance quality, and timeliness may be appropriate. Targets for the number of various activities to be carried out may also be useful in describing the expected programme efforts. Outcome targets will be useful in describing reductions in the occurrence of disease or disease complications. However, such targets may be of limited value in reflecting the effect of the intervention activities because the surveillance system prior to intervention will have usually underestimated the occurrence of disease and of complications. An alternative approach is to estimate the number of averted cases and/or complications.

## 14.3 Specify and procure resources

Particular attention must be given to ensuring that the required resources are available. On the basis of the estimates of resources needed and the proportion of these that are or will be available, the manager can estimate the type and amount of resources still required. This listing will then become the starting point for efforts to obtain the resources. Many different sources of funds should be considered, both within the country and abroad. Within the country, other ministry of health programmes, e.g., primary health care, maternal and child health, and family planning, may be able to provide resources for control activities associated with sexually transmitted diseases when these are shown to enhance the efficacity of their own programme. Resources from the ministries of education or of rural development may also be available when such activities reflect their goals. Non-governmental sources such as mission groups, women's organizations, and voluntary funds should also be considered. Finally, community organizations may provide the necessary funds when these resources will directly benefit the community group. External resources may be available from health and non-health organizations through bilateral arrangements or from international organizations such as UNFPA, UNICEF, WHO, IPPF, and others. These potential resource donors should be considered and requests made to the specific group(s) most likely to provide the necessary support.

## 14.4 Develop a work system

The functions necessary to carry out the interventions can be formulated on the basis of the strategy designs. Functions that should generally be included are: secure, train, and supervise personnel; obtain materials; provide for transportation; ensure maintenance of equipment;

evaluate the programme; and perform research. However, the details of the functions depend upon the design of the particular strategies.

An overall management system can then be developed, assigning the required functions to particular individuals and providing for the coordination and supervision of these personnel. With an overall system design, it is possible to describe each job responsibility, taking into consideration the qualifications, training, supervision, and evaluation required for each.

The overall work system is one way of planning for programme management. Other, less formal, methods may also be useful under different circumstances.

## 14.5 General principles

*Programme manager*

To ensure that all the many aspects of the control programme are coordinated effectively, it is necessary to appoint an overall manager with the responsibility and authority to make changes. This may be a full-time position devoted exclusively to the control programme or sexually transmitted diseases may be one of several disease problems covered by a more comprehensive managerial position. The most important qualities of the manager will be his personality, management skills, and interest in the job. Although important, relevant experience with sexually transmitted diseases and clinical, microbiological, or epidemiological skills may be less important to success of the programme.

*Approaches to change*

The manager will develop the methods necessary for making any changes by considering and applying whatever alternative approaches are available. The approaches for inducing change include: the rational approach; the "train-a-trainer" approach; or the model or demonstration approach (*1*).

(1) *Rational approach.* The rational approach is useful when there is little resistance to change. In particular, this approach can reinforce cooperation between persons who are already interested. Thus, it will be most useful for health providers who have had some experience with sexually transmitted diseases, selected university staff or other professionals, and community groups where the consequences of these diseases have become apparent.

(2) *Train-a-trainer.* The "train-a-trainer" approach involves working with a small group of individuals. After intensive training, these individuals then train further trainers or actually train the audience. For instance, senior personnel in the control programme should be training teachers, university lecturers, nurses, and other health personnel. Once trained, these personnel should be able subsequently to train or educate others. The

training approach, however, can also be used to encourage broader social changes that are helpful to the programme. Training key opinion and organizational leaders in appropriate aspects of the programme should encourage them to adopt control of sexually transmitted diseases as one of their own activities of interest. This approach can be one of the most efficient and inexpensive methods of inducing social change.

(3) *Model approach*. The model or demonstration approach provides a practical example to individuals. Individuals learn how to operate or conduct an activity by observing it in action; thus, the activity is clarified and its function is emphasized. This approach is very persuasive, and therefore, may be of particular value for individuals who resist change. The model approach is also useful when attempting to introduce highly innovative ideas or activities requiring extensive integration. In such settings it may be difficult, even for the enthusiastic, to appreciate fully the nuances of new concepts or the complex interaction of the components of a programme.

*Inducing change*

Special attention should be paid to two general groups: decision-makers and first-line workers. Decision-makers are generally receptive to those changes which reinforce their authority or enlarge their influence. They will be most interested in the planning and organization of the intervention. They will avoid areas of change associated with potentially adverse political ramifications. First-line workers are generally opposed to change, because they are overworked. The existing work-load may prevent them from learning new methods. In addition, because of work stress they may be unable to envisage the potential benefits of any changes made. Finally, plans for change often do not reflect the current interests or future needs of these workers.

To induce change with decision-makers, quantitative information, an overview of the programme effects, and examples of success of the programme elsewhere may be most useful. Decision-makers will also wish to influence the change manner in which directions are given so that the changes made become their own.

First-line workers need to be involved in the planning for change (2). The programme manager must also recognize the increased need for supervisory involvement during the change period to facilitate the transition. Methods for fostering peer approval should be sought, including group meetings where recognition of desired behaviour and information exchange are emphasized. Periodic newsletters, or other forms of written feedback with circulation to the entire group can emphasize the same topics. Whenever possible, these workers should be encouraged to express their point of view, particularly as the details of their new activities are developed. Such personnel should also be involved in developing methods to evaluate these activities. In addition, they must be given the opportunity to understand the overall programme efforts in order to clarify their contribution to the programme.

*Coordination*

All control programmes should have clearly understood lines of authority and supervisory responsibility. Daily management functions should be delegated by the manager to leaders of subunits within the organization. However, the programme manager has overall responsibility for management and must develop efficient communication channels to ensure that all the required information can move rapidly from him to each individual, and vice versa. This can be achieved by regular meetings between the manager and unit leaders and between unit leaders and the people in each unit. Provision should also be made for periodic meetings between the manager and each employee. Such a system provides more personalized communication than written material. However, important guidelines or policies should also be provided to all staff in written form to ensure their accurate transmittal. In very large organizations, there should be a mechanism for ensuring that all staff have seen such guidelines or policy documents.

## 14.6 Summary

No standard approach to the organization and management of a control programme is appropriate for all settings. The problems, the sociocultural milieu, and the resources will be unique to each country. Programme management must consider the variety of opportunities available and develop a plan for effecting change. In general, programme changes or new programmes should begin in the area and with the problem where there is the greatest chance of success. When success has been demonstrated, the programme can be more readily expanded. An overall work system should be developed which will assist in ensuring that the wide variety of necessary activities are implemented in a coordinated fashion.

### References

1. LEWIN, K. Group decisions and social change. In: Newcomb, T. M. et al. *Readings in social psychology.* New York, Henry Holt and Company, 1947.
2. McMAHON, R. ET AL. *On being in charge. A guide for middle-level management in primary health care.* Geneva, World Health Organization, 1980.

# Chapter 15. Evaluation of control programmes

## 15.1 Introduction

Evaluation is the process by which results are compared with the intended objectives, or more simply the assessment of how well a programme is performing. When evaluating a programme it is not only necessary to determine whether the expected results were obtained, but also to verify that these results were a consequence of the programme activities. This last requirement of "causality" makes evaluation a complex and difficult task and means that evaluation must be divided into different types, levels, and approaches (see below).

*Purposes of evaluation*

Since the merits of a programme or activity are being assessed by evaluation (*1*, *2*), the exact aims of the evaluation must be decided before the process begins. Evaluations are undertaken to assist in making decisions regarding the programme: whether it should be initiated, continued, changed, or improved. Activities carried out to justify decisions already made or simply to record that an evaluation has taken place will not be considered in this chapter.

*Types of evaluation*

There are several different types of evaluation applicable to control programmes for sexually transmitted diseases (*3*, *4*) (see Table 6):

(1) *Front-end or feasibility analysis* encompasses those evaluation activities that take place prior to the initiation of a programme. These analyses provide guidance for refining programme plans, determining the appropriate level of implementation effort, and deciding whether to begin the programme at all. This type of evaluation should be part of the initial planning for the programme (Chapter 2).

(2) *Evaluation assessment* attempts to clarify whether a programme could be evaluated if implemented. Often, programmes cannot be evaluated because their objectives are not clear or necessary data are not available. If a programme cannot be evaluated, a first step would be to reformulate or redefine the objectives and identify possible sources of usable data.

(3) *Programme monitoring* is the most common form of evaluation; it varies from periodic checks of compliance with policies and procedures to the relatively straightforward "tracking" of services delivered, and "counting" of clients.

**Table 6. Health programme evaluations: considerations and characteristics**

| Purpose | Type of evaluation | Approach | Focus of evaluation | Sources of data | User(s) of the information | Degree of difficulty to perform |
|---|---|---|---|---|---|---|
| To quantify activities and services provided | Programme monitoring | Economic | Productivity of programme (process; outputs) | Records of activities | Managers, administrators | + |
| To assess efficiency of programme or its components | Programme monitoring | Economic | Utilization of resources (inputs, process, and outputs) | Records of activities, accounting data | Administrators, managers, health planners | + + |
| To assess quality of services | Programme monitoring, formative evaluation | Economic and health benefit | Quality of care (input, process, outputs, and outcomes) | Record audit; direct observation of medical process; patient or provider questionnaire | Health providers, educators, administrators, policy-makers | + + + |
| To determine health benefits for target populations | Summative, formative evaluations | Economic, health benefit (societal) | Benefits of programme (outcomes) | Routine health statistics, appropriate surveys | Planners, policy-makers, researchers | + + + |

(4) *Formative evaluations* are carried out during the programme so that the results can be immediately used to make any necessary changes.

(5) *Summative evaluations* are those which retrospectively assess the programme after completion, or at predetermined points during its implementation.

Ideally, all these types of evaluation should be incorporated into a control programme. In reality, this is seldom done, and most policy makers and administrators are satisfied with programme monitoring or with partial summative evaluations of the programme.

## Approaches to evaluation

Whatever the type of evaluation used, and depending on the concerns of the user and the intended uses of the information, three approaches to programme evaluation are feasible:

(1) *Economic approaches* place the major emphasis on the programme efficiency. For example, screening more patients in a given time or at a lower cost would be valued most highly;

(2) *Health benefit approaches* focus on the health improvements that result from various strategies or activities and those which give the greatest health benefit would be valued most highly. The benefits considered in this approach are not only those obtained under optimal conditions (efficacy), but also those obtained under normal field use (effectiveness);

(3) *Societal approaches* combine the economic and health benefit approaches in a broader, more complex analysis of the programme. Such an approach attempts to compare the social benefits of the programme with those of other health and social programmes that are competing for the same scarce resources. Traditionally, control programmes in many settings have not had an appropriate share of the overall health budget, therefore this approach may be particularly important.

Both cost-benefit analysis (CBA) and cost-effectiveness analysis (CEA) (5, 6), assume that since health resources are limited, it is necessary to extract the maximum benefit from the money spent. In CBA the costs of a particular course of action are measured in monetary terms and weighed against the benefits derived, which are also measured in monetary values. The action will be implemented if the financial benefits are greater than the costs. However, there is disagreement not only on the methods to be used for monetary valuation but also on the advisability or feasibility of assigning monetary values to such intangible items as patient suffering and social or family disruption which occurs because of sexually transmitted diseases. CEA avoids these difficult problems by relating the costs of different strategies or programmes with various benefits such as averted fetal deaths or avoided hospitalizations or surgery for pelvic inflammatory disease, without converting these benefits into monetary terms. Both CBA and CEA are difficult to carry out. The variables that need to be measured include the long-term morbidity of sexually transmitted disease and the associated costs to individuals, their families, and society.

## Levels of evaluation

A health programme is basically a system (7) in which the programme resources (inputs) are used (processes) to perform activities (output) resulting in an improvement in the health of the population (outcomes) (Fig. 2). Thus, the personnel, materials, and organizational structures of the programme are used to achieve certain ends such as diagnosing and treating patients, performing laboratory tests, or identifying sexual partners. As a result of these interactions, disease complications will be prevented and disease transmission will be decreased. The requisites for evaluation at each of these points in the system are the availability of reliable and valid ways of measuring them.

**Fig. 2.   The health programme system**

| INPUTS | PROCESSES | OUTPUTS | OUTCOMES |
|---|---|---|---|

Structure of organization
Administration
Facilities
Equipment
Personnel
Supplies

Programme activities

Use of services
Volume of activities

Impact on:
morbidity
mortality
sequelae
consequences
patient satisfaction

WHO 84484

## 15.2. Principles for the evaluation of control programmes

### Evaluation of the programme or its components

Ideally, the whole programme should be evaluated; however, in many instances only isolated components can be assessed. Furthermore, evaluations of control programmes for sexually transmitted diseases range from assessment at the national level to the more modest and feasible assessment of clinical services or other programme components at regional or local levels.

Control programmes vary in structure and function in different settings. In countries with categorical programmes, the manager has knowledge of and control over both inputs and processes, and can assess the outputs and outcomes of his programme. In most countries, the components of the control programme are shared with other programmes; the manager has only partial knowledge and control over the shared components. In these situations, evaluation is much more difficult. A third, common type of control programme is where the manager has little control over the inputs that filter through a maze of loosely organized components. In such an integrated programme, evaluation may be unrewarding because the manager can only assess parts of some of the programme components and has limited authority to make changes. This situation may lead to poor planning, inefficiency, and ineffectiveness of the control programme.

## Orientation of evaluation

The health systems approach is based on the premise that "good" inputs will lead to "good" processes, and hence to "good" outcomes. A practical approach is to assess the part of the system for which reliable data are available or can be obtained. Although it is most desirable to measure and evaluate the outcomes (health benefits) of the control programme in the community, the absence of reliable baseline data may preclude this type of assessment in many settings. Therefore, in most countries, control evaluation efforts focus on structure and process rather than outcome. In a few countries, where control programmes are well-developed and good information and data systems exist, the more complex evaluations of outcome assessments are possible.

## Uses and purposes of evaluation

Evaluation must be an integral part of the control process and provide continuous feedback to the programme. Systems to monitor programme implementation and the efficiency, effectiveness, and impact of a programme operate at two interconnected levels, the policy and the managerial levels. Policy-makers will be most interested in outcome evaluations to determine whether there has been any progress in the control of sexually transmitted diseases and if the policies, strategies, or plans of action need to be revised. On the other hand, managers will be particularly interested in evaluations of the day-to-day processes. These evaluations will reveal whether the necessary services and their support activities are developed and efficient. Such assessments can result in prompt programme corrections.

## Planning and implementing the evaluation

Specific mention of evaluations relating to some of the strategies and support services has been made in preceeding chapters. As an example of the process of evaluation, the evaluation of clinical services includes assessment of the quality and quantity and results in the establishment of an ongoing system to ensure that the necessary standards are being met (quality assurance). The sequence of evaluation activities includes:

(1) *Define the objectives.* An important issue or activity which warrants evaluation must be identified and the objectives of such a focus should be

clarified. This can be done by canvassing personnel or patients, reviewing clinic documents, or observing clinic activities. From this identification, an objective can be developed and clarified with staff. This process must also reflect the ultimate purpose of the evaluation; in this case, to effect change.

(2) *Clarify the methods.* The level of evaluation and the data to be collected need to be considered so that the methods of measurement reflect the intended uses of the evaluation. For example, the data collected might include personnel numbers and types, space, and materials, and contrast these data to the number of patients, their sex distribution and the type of problem, if the evaluation was intended to emphasize the need for greater resources.

(3) *Specify criteria for the expected standards.* It will be necessary to develop explicit criteria of what constitutes the standard of quality. This may be done by asking "experts." Alternatively, if resources are the focus, criteria used in other clinical services may be applied.

(4) *Identify data units.* Develop a way to identify possible units of study so that comparisons can be made. For example, routine examinations of men and women require different amounts of time, expertise, and resources. Complex problems require more tests and evaluation time than routine attendance, etc.

(5) *Define the amount of data needed.* The amount of data required will depend on the purpose and use of the evaluation. An end-point to data collection should be selected, based on the time period or quantity of data needed.

(6) *Collect and analyse the data.* Carry out the evaluation and assess the results.

(7) *Use the data.* This information must be presented to the target audience in order to begin corrective actions. The identified deficiencies may be directly altered by the target group, or they may ensure that the necessary changes are made. An ongoing system of evaluation may be established for some types of issues. For example, continuous assessment of the clinical services quality can be encouraged by a quality assurance programme of continuous data collection, analysis, and feedback.

## 15.3 Evaluation of control.

Evaluation should always be considered during the planning and implementation stages of a programme or activity. Evaluation is important for the continuous monitoring of programme activities and may be crucial in identifying the health benefits derived. Furthermore, even in such a well-developed control programme for sexually transmitted diseases as that established in the United Kingdom, evaluations can be useful in identifying performance difficulties (8, 9). Evaluation studies may also be carried out to generate information for other purposes. Examples of these other uses of evaluations of control programmes for sexually transmitted diseases are given in Annex 5.

# References

1. WORLD HEALTH ORGANIZATION. *Health programme evaluation*. Geneva, WHO, 1981 ("Health for All" Series, No. 6).
2. SHORTELL, S. M. & RICHARDSON, C. B. *Health program evaluation*. St. Louis, Mosby Company, 1978.
3. RUTMAN, L. *Evaluation research methods: A basic guide*. Beverly Hills, Sage Publications, 1977.
4. EVALUATION RESEARCH SOCIETY. *Standards for program evaluation*. Mimeograph exposive draft, San Francisco, 1980.
5. THOMPSON, M. S. *Benefit-cost analysis for program evaluation*. Beverly Hills, Sage Publications, 1980.
6. WARNER, K. E. & HUTTON, R. C. Cost-benefit and cost-effectiveness analysis in health care. *Medical care*, **18**: 1069–1984 (1980).
7. REISMAN, A. *Systems analysis in health-care delivery*. Lexington, Lexington Books, 1979.
8. ADLER, M. W. ET AL. Facilities and diagnostic criteria in sexually transmitted disease clinics in England and Wales. *British journal of venereal diseases*, **54**: 2–9 (1978).
9. ADLER, M. W. ET AL. Sexually transmitted diseases in a defined population of women. *British medical journal*, **2**: 29–32 (1981).

# Annex 1. Tests available for the early detection of sexually transmitted diseases

The tests most frequently used for the early detection of disease are syphilis serology, wet-mount microscopy (vaginal secretions), or Gram-stained smears (urethral, cervical secretions) and cultures of the responsible organism (*Neisseria gonorrhoeae, Chlamydia trachomatis,* etc.) A brief discussion follows on some tests currently used for the detection of syphilis and gonorrhoea, the two diseases traditionally included in most control programmes. In general, as culture tests for *N. gonorrhoeae* become available, they should first be used for (early) diagnosis in symptomatic patients, particularly females, in order to improve the management of those cases and their sexual contacts (*1*). Syphilis serological tests should be used mainly for diagnosis in symptomatic patients and in case-finding programmes among pregnant women where disease prevalence is high.

## 1. Tests used in gonorrhoea screening and case-finding

*Gram stain*

This test is easy to use, generally available, inexpensive, and specific. The specificity varies according to the site from which the specimen is obtained: for example, whether it is from high in the urethra or low in the cervix. In men with abundant urethral discharge and women with abundant cervical discharge, the test is sensitive, but in asymptomatic males and females the sensitivity is approximately 60% (*2*). Again, the concept of predictive value is extremely important in this regard. If we assume that a Gram-stained cervical smear for the diagnosis of gonorrhoea in females has a 50% sensitivity and 90% specificity, the predictive value of a positive smear at a 15% prevalence rate of gonorrhoea is 47%. In this example, the prevalence of gonorrhoea is high, and a good validity of the Gram-stained cervical smear is presumed; however, this test is not suitable in non-selective programmes for the early detection of gonorrhoea in females.

*Indirect fluorescent antibody test (IFAT)*

IFAT has aproximately the same specificity as Gram staining but is more sensitive. It is expensive to set up, requires specially trained personnel, and is usually available only at the central level. Consequently, it is not commonly used in gonorrhoea screening programmes.

*Culture methods*

When primary isolation is followed by *Neisseria* species identification through sugar utilization tests, there is 100% specificity with specimens taken from any site. This is especially important when screening homosexual anal specimens and any pharyngeal specimen where differentiation from *N. meningitidis* must be achieved (2, 3). When sugar utilization tests are not done, only cultures from cervical and urethral sites are highly specific.

With or without specific identification of the organism, gonorrhoea cultures are very sensitive in mildly symptomatic and asymptomatic females and males. Because of this, cultures are the only recommended test for gonorrhoea screening and case-finding at present.

Culture screening is almost prohibitively expensive in some countries, and in addition may not be technically feasible in some settings. In many countries, bacteriological laboratory facilities are available for only a small proportion of the population. The use of transport media may increase the population that can be covered, but it also increases the culture costs and may adversely affect the culture sensitivity.

The use of both cultures and slide methods requires genital examination, and this is not acceptable to many population groups, particularly when used for screening purposes. Culture of the first-void urine (FVU) for selective screening of males may overcome the acceptance problems in this group (4, 5). This procedure has not been extensively evaluated and could only be used in programmes with good laboratory support.

*Serology*

Serological tests based on the presence of antibody to gonococcal antigens may in the future become an important epidemiological tool (6). However, at present, serological tests are only at the research stage. Sensitivity and specificity must be increased before serology becomes potentially useful for mass gonorrhoea screening programmes (7, 8). Serological tests are not useful for early detection because positive tests indicate present as well as past infections and there is a cross reaction with other species of *Neisseria* (8).

For the present, if screening and case-finding programmes for gonorrhoea are contemplated, they must be based on the use of the culture test.

## 2. Tests used in syphilis screening and case-finding

Screening and case-finding are much more feasible for syphilis than they are for gonorrhoea. The tests (e.g., RPR card test and VDRL slide test) are sensitive, specific, reliable, acceptable, and generally available. In addition, the long natural history of the disease and its self-limitation as regards transmission increase the effectiveness of detection programmes.

Serological screening for syphilis is often based on the use of several different serological tests in series to enhance the test specificity. A reagin test such as the VDRL test is carried out first; this test is highly sensitive for the detection of "active" syphilis, and it is followed by a treponemal test that is more specific, such as the TPHA or the FTA-ABS.

*Reagin tests (non-treponemal)*

(a) *Venereal disease research laboratory (VDRL) test.* The VDRL test is sensitive for early syphilis. Quantitative tests reveal rapid decreases in antibody titre following the treatment of early syphilis such that most patients become seronegative within a year (9). Although false positive results may occur in patients with certain infectious and non-infectious diseases (10), the VDRL test specificity using commercial antigens is less than 1% (11).

(b) *Rapid plasma-reagin card test (RPR).* This screening test uses a stabilized VDRL antigen with attached charcoal particles. The flocculation reaction can be read without a microscope, provides results within 4 minutes, and can use plasma separated from finger-prick specimens. Thus, the RPR is practical for screening in settings where there are no elaborate laboratory facilities. In some countries, other non-treponemal tests such as the Wassermann test are still being used, but these are being progressively replaced by the VDRL and RPR tests.

*Treponemal tests*

(a) *Treponema pallidum immobilization test (TPI).* The TPI test is the standard against which all treponemal tests are compared. It is a research tool and is never used for screening.

(b) *Fluorescent treponemal antibody absorption test (FTA-ABS).* FTA-ABS combines high sensitivity for early syphilis, as well as all other stages, with high specificity. It is used mostly to confirm positive non-treponemal (reagin) tests.

(c) *Haemagglutination treponemal tests.* There is no consensus on the sensitivity and advantages of several haemagglutination tests (11–13), but this test procedure is increasingly replacing the FTA-ABS as a confirmation test. In late disease, it is more sensitive than the non-treponemal tests, and this coupled with its low cost and technical feasibility have led some to suggest that it should be used for screening and case-finding (13).

## 3. Tests used for screening and case-finding of other sexually transmitted diseases

Chlamydial infections due to serotypes D–K are possibly the most frequent and perhaps the most important sexually transmitted disease in developed countries (14–17). Chlamydial case-finding has been considered for pregnant women (15), women attending clinics (17), and other high-risk groups such as prostitutes (18).

Tests available include cell cultures, slide methods (Giemsa staining and fluorescent antibody) and serological tests (microimmunofluorescence test). At present, only cell cultures are particularly useful for early detection programmes for *Chlamydia trachomatis.* Case-finding by culturing for *C. trachomatis* in high-risk individuals has been recommended (16). However, for most countries early detection programmes for *C. trachomatis* infections are not realistic because of the costs involved and the unavailability of adequate laboratory facilities.

However, new test technologies are being rapidly developed, based on the development and use of monoclonal antibodies (*19*). This and other non-culture methods (*20*) will result in dramatic changes in the procedures available for case-finding and screening.

## References

1. WHITBY, G. L. Screening for disease, definition and criteria. *Lancet*, **2**: 819–821 (1974).
2. WHO Technical Report Series, No. 616, 1978 (Neisseria gonorrhoeae *and gonococcal infections*: report of a WHO Scientific Group).
3. FAUR, Y. C. ET AL. Isolation of *N. meningitidis* from patients in a gonorrhoea screening program. A four year survey in New York City. *American journal of public health*, **71**: 53–58. (1981).
4. MURRAY, E. S. ET AL. Options for diagnosis and control of gonorrheal urethritis in males using uncentrifuged voided urine (FVU) as a specimen for culture. *American journal of public health*, **69**: 596–598 (1979).
5. LUCIANO, A. A. & GRUBIN, L. Gonorrhoea screening. Comparison of three techniques. *Journal of the American Medical Association*, **243**: 680–681 (1980).
6. QUIGLEY, M. M. Place for gonorrhoea serology. *New York journal of medicine*, **77**: 2053–2055 (1977).
7. WILLIAMS, R. P. & CHILDRESS, J. R. Variation in responses to four serological tests for gonorrhoea. In: Brooks, G. F. et al., ed. *Immune biology of* Neisseria gonorrhoeae. Washington, DC, American Society for Microbiology, 1978, pp. 382–384.
8. HOLMES, K. K. ET AL. Is serology useful in gonorrhoea? A critical analysis of factors influencing serodiagnosis. In: Brooks, G. F. et al., ed. *Immune biology of* Neisseria gonorrhoeae. Washington, DC, American Society for Microbiology, 1978, pp. 370–376.
9. SPARLING, P. F. Diagnosis and treatment of syphilis. *New England journal of medicine*, **284**: 642–653 (1971).
10. TRAMONT, E. C. *Treponema pallidum* (syphilis). In: Mandell, G. L. et al., ed. *Principles and practice of infectious diseases*. New York, John Wiley & Sons, 1979.
11. JAFFE, H. W. ET AL. Hemagglutination tests for syphilis antibody. *American journal clinical pathology*, **70**: 230–233 (1978).
12. MACFARLANE, D. E. & ELIAS-JONES, T. F. Screening tests for syphilis. A comparison of the Treponema pallidum hemagglutination assay with two automated serological tests. *British journal of venereal diseases*, **53**: 348–352 (1977).
13. LUGER, A. ET AL. Specificity of the *Treponema pallidum* haemagglutination test-analysis of results. *British journal of venereal diseases*, (1981).
14. SCHACHTER, J. Editorial–The expanding clinical spectrum of infections with *C. trachomatis*. *Sexually transmitted diseases*, **4**: 116–118 (1977).
15. SCHACHTER, J. & GROSSMAN, M. Chlamydial infections. *Annual review of medicine*, **32**: 45–61 (1981).
16. HANDSFIELD, H. H. ET AL. Public health implications and control of sexually transmitted chlamydial infections. *Sexually transmitted diseases*, **8**: 85–86 (1981).
17. RICHMOND, S. J. ET AL. Value and feasibility of screening women attending STD clinics for cervical chlamydial infections. *British journal of venereal diseases*, **56**: 92–95 (1980).
18. REEVES, W. C. ET AL. Epidemiología de las enfermedades transmitidas sexualmente en un grupo de mujeres de alto riesgo en Panamá. *Revista médica de Panamá*, **5**: 209–222 (1980).
19. NOWINSKI, R.C. ET AL. Monoclonal antibodies for diagnosis of infectious diseases in humans. *Science*, **219**: 637–644 (1983).
20. JAFFE, H. W. ET AL. Diagnosis of gonorrhoea using a genetic transformation test on mailed clinical specimens. *Journal of infectious diseases*, **146**: 275–279 (1982).

# Annex 2. Prototype patient care protocol: urethral discharge[1]

## 1. Background

Males frequently attend health care facilities with complaints of urethral discharge, dysuria, or frequency of micturition. When the patient is examined, the health worker may find: a yellow or clear/white urethral discharge, a purulent preputial discharge associated with ulcerations, or no discharge (2).

## 2. Data needed

In each country a protocol can be empirically chosen, implemented, and subsequently evaluated. Its effectiveness can be considerably improved if data are collected before and at regular intervals during implementation. This data could include: frequency of gonococcal infections, as determined by Gram-stained smears of urethral discharge; frequency of *N. gonorrhoeae* infection (and nongonococcal infection) as determined by culture of urethral discharge; antibiotic susceptibility patterns of gonococci and the prevalence of penicillinase-producing gonococci (PPNG); and results of clinical trials of several different treatment regimens considered for use in the protocol. For example, in Swaziland the etiology of urethral discharge was studied twice (3, 4). In January 1978, 82% of patients with urethral discharge had gonorrhoea, and 18% had either nongonococcal urethritis (NGU) or no urethritis. When repeated in January 1979, of 98 patients with urethral discharge, 88% had gonorrhoea, 5% had NGU, and 7% had no urethritis. Only 1.4% of gonorrhoea patients were also infected with *C. trachomatis*. Of the 70 gonococcal strains tested, none was PPNG; 51% were highly sensitive to penicillin (MIC: $\leqslant 0.06\,\mu g/ml$), 18% had slightly diminished sensitivity (MIC: between $0.06$–$0.25\,\mu g/ml$), and 31% were even less sensitive (MIC $\geqslant 0.5\,\mu g/ml$).[2] No strain had a MIC greater than $1\,\mu g/ml$ for tetracycline. Based on these *in vitro* susceptibilities, a 6% failure rate was predicted for the APPG (aqueous procaine penicillin G) plus probenecid regimen (5).

## 3. Patient care strategy (protocol design)

Based on the above data, the following strategy was devised for the management of males with urethritis in Swaziland. If no discharge is seen the patient is asked to return the following morning before urinating. If, however, a urethral discharge is seen the procedure is as shown in Fig. 3. The underlying rationale is that all urethral discharge is considered to be

---

[1] Adapted from Meheus (1).
[2] MIC = minimal inhibitory concentration.

## Fig. 3. Urethral discharge protocol

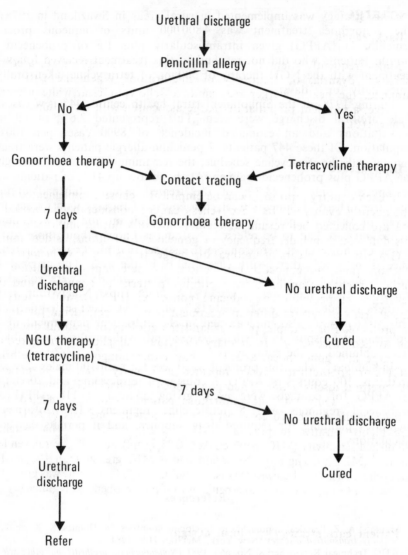

gonorrhoea, and that it should be treated with an antibiotic, preferably in a single dose. Contacts of the patient are traced and receive the same treatment. At the one-week follow-up visit, those patients who have not responded to the initial therapy receive a treatment which is effective against both potentially uncured gonococcal urethritis and nongonococcal urethritis (NGU).

## 4. Experience

This strategy was implemented in rural areas in Swaziland in 1978 *(4)*. The gonorrhoea treatment was 4 800 000 units of aqueous procaine penicillin G (APPG) given intramuscularly plus 1 g of probenecid by mouth. Patients who did not respond to this treatment received follow-up treatment with the NGU therapy of 500 mg of tetracycline taken orally 4 times daily for 7 days.

During 1978, at the Siphofaneni rural health centre, 447 new cases of male urethral discharge were seen. This represented 2.6% of all new consultations and an estimated incidence of 8900 cases per 100 000 population. Of these 447 patients, 7 penicillin-allergic patients were treated initially with the tetracycline schedule; the remaining 440 patients were given the APPG plus probenecid regimen. At the follow-up 41% of patients were present and only 21 (4.7% of the treated group) still had urethral discharge. These 21 patients received a course of therapy with tetracycline. Seven of these 21 patients returned for follow-up and all were cured. Hence, no case had to be referred. Nothing is known about those lost to follow-up; however, it is reasonable to assume that most cases were cured since there is no other health care facility in the area. The original 447 patients mentioned 534 sexual partners; since only 192 were considered traceable, these men were given 192 contact slips. Ninety-four sexual partners attended and were treated (18% of the 534 recent sexual partners). This strategy was also implemented in the outpatient department of the Government Hospital in Mbabane, Swaziland, with results comparable to those obtained in the rural areas.

In summary, when this protocol was used, for each 100 males seen with urethritis, 100 courses of APPG, 6 courses of tetracycline, and 20 courses of APPG for contacts were used, giving a total of 118 APPG and probenecid regimens and 8 tetracycline regimens. This information facilitates planning for required drug supplies, and it permits easy cost calculations.

## References

1. MEHEUS, A. Z. Practical approaches in developing countries. In: Holmes, K. K. et al., ed. *Sexually transmitted diseases.* New York, McGraw-Hill, 1984.
2. WHO Technical Report Series, No. 660, 1981 (*Nongonococcal urethritis and other selected sexually transmitted diseases of public health importance:* report of a WHO Scientific Group).
3. MEHEUS, A. ET AL. Genital infections in Swaziland. *Annales de la Société belge de médecine tropicale,* **62**: 361–367 (1982).
4. MEHEUS, A. ET AL. Epidemiology and aetiology of urethritis in Swaziland. *International journal of epidemiology,* **9**: 239–245 (1980).
5. JAFFE, H. W. ET AL. National gonorrhoea therapy monitoring study. *In vitro* antibiotic susceptibility and its correlation with treatment results. *New England journal of medicine,* **294**: 5–9 (1976).

# Annex 3. Prototype patient care protocol: vaginal discharge[1]

## 1. Background

Women frequently attend health facilities with complaints of abnormal vaginal discharge, dysuria, vulvar itching, and lower abdominal pain. The health care provider must differentiate between lower genital tract infections, pelvic inflammatory disease (PID), and other medical or surgical conditions unrelated to sexually transmitted diseases.

If pelvic inflammatory disease (PID) is suspected, the patient should be referred to a well-equipped clinic. However, when this is impossible, the health worker must distinguish this condition from others, particularly those requiring surgery, using general patient management suggestions for lower abdominal pain (2). When immediate surgical intervention is not indicated, the diagnosis can be made by finding bilateral lower abdominal pain, mucopurulent cervical discharge, abnormal tenderness on bimanual pelvic examination, pain on motion of the cervix, and fever. A typical treatment for PID is 500 mg of tetracycline hydrochloride given orally 4 times daily for 10 days. Sexual partner(s) should receive the same tetracycline regimen for 7 days, even if they have no symptoms.

## 2. Data needed

Information useful to the development of a vaginal discharge protocol includes identification of the common agents associated with this problem. In Africa (Table 7) patients complaining of vaginal discharge frequently have gonococcal infection (3, 4). Since the prevalence of gonorrhoea is based on a single cervical culture (sensitivity 80–90 %), the "true" prevalence is more likely to be between 20 and 35 % (5).

Table 7. Microorganisms isolated from cervical or vaginal specimens from patients from Kenya and Swaziland who complained of vaginal discharge

| Species | Percentage positive | |
| --- | --- | --- |
| | Mbabane, Swaziland (n = 65) | Nairobi, Kenya (n = 54) |
| Neisseria gonorrhoeae | 21.5 | 30.0 |
| Trichomonas vaginalis | 24.6 | 31.5 |
| Candida albicans | 23.1 | 14.5 |
| Gardnerella vaginalis | NT[a] | 69.0 |

[a] NT = not tested.

[1] Adapted from Meheus (1)

## Fig. 4. Vaginal discharge protocol

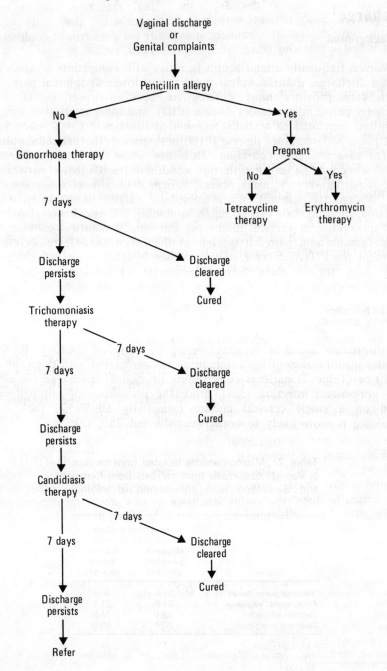

Where the prevalence of gonococcal infection is 20% or more among patients with vaginal discharge, the initial treatment should be for gonorrhoea. Since patients with vaginal discharge are almost always given symptomatic treatment, treatment specifically for gonorrhoea could even be considered where the gonorrhoea prevalence is below 20%.

## 3. Patient care strategy

After managing surgical patients and patients with pelvic inflammatory disease, the remaining women with genital complaints should be examined to identify those with ulcers. Then, regardless of the presence of vaginal discharge, all such women should receive treatment for gonorrhoea (Fig. 4). If the patient has not improved within a week the genitalia should be reinspected. Those patients having objective vaginal discharge would then receive treatment for trichomoniasis, i.e., metronidazole in a single oral dose of 2 g. The patient should be advised to return in one week if symptoms persist. If objective vaginal discharge is still present, antimycotic vaginal tablets should be given. If complaints continue, then the patient should be referred to a more specialized facility.

## 4. Experience

This strategy was implemented in a rural health centre in Swaziland in 1978. During one year, 316 new cases of vaginal discharge were seen, representing 1.9% of all new consultations. These patients initially received the APPG and probenecid therapy for gonorrhoea. At the first follow-up visit 38% were still symptomatic and therefore received treatment for trichomoniasis. At the second follow-up, 4% attended and received treatment for candidiasis; 1% finally had to be referred because symptoms persisted despite the treatments given.

This simplified approach to vaginal discharge is far from perfect. However, in many developing countries, health workers frequently encounter this clinical problem. Without recommendations, these workers may refuse to dispense treatment or may select a treatment regimen that is inadequate, e.g., sulfadimidine, for virtually all common agents (6).

## References

1. MEHEUS. A. Z. Practical approaches in developing countries. In: Holmes, K. K. et al., ed. *Sexually transmitted diseases.* New York, McGraw-Hill, 1984.
2. *The primary health worker* (revised edition). Geneva, World Health Organization, 1980.
3. MEHEUS, A. ET AL. Genital infections in Swaziland. *Annales de la Société belge de médecine tropicale,* 62: 361–367 (1982).
4. PIOT, P. *Gardnerella vaginalis* and *Gardnerella*-associated vaginitis. Ph. D. Thesis, University of Antwerp (UIA), 1981.

5. OSOBA, A. O. Epidemiology of urethritis in Ibadan. *British journal of venereal diseases,* **48**: 116–120 (1972).
6. ARYA, O. P. & BENNETT, F. J. The use and misuse of medicines in relation to some sexually transmitted diseases in Uganda. In: Bagshawe, A. F. et al., ed. *The use and abuse of drugs in tropical Africa.* Nairobi, East African Literature Bureau, 1974.

# Annex 4. Prototype patient care protocol: genital ulcers[1]

## 1. Background

Genital ulcers may be infectious, resulting from syphilis, chancroid, herpes, lymphogranuloma venereum, and donovanosis, or non-infectious and mainly traumatic. Careful clinical examination is the first, most important, and frequently the only diagnostic tool for the evaluation of genital ulcers (2–5). Genital ulcers do not usually correspond to the "typical" textbook description. As a result, the diagnosis of genital ulcers is often incorrect and their management is ineffective. As many as 30–50% of primary syphilis lesions are atypical (the chancre is painful, not indurated or multiple) (6). Herpes simplex virus (HSV) infection combined with poor genital hygiene can result in multiple, soft, superinfected, very painful genital ulcers resembling chancroid (45% of herpes cases in a study in Swaziland were clinically diagnosed as chancroid) (7). In the United States of America the accuracy of clinical diagnosis was also quite poor for lesions due to *T. pallidum* (78%), *Herpes virus hominis* (63%), and *Haemophilus ducreyi* (33%) (8).

A microbiological diagnosis of genital ulcers is valuable because it then becomes possible to provide specific treatment to patients and sexual partners. The cost-efficiency of these tests must, however, be evaluated if they are intended to guide patient care. When resources and facilities become available, the first tests to be added to the clinical diagnosis should be dark-field microscopy and a qualitative and quantitative reagin test (2).

## 2. Data needed

There are major differences in the etiology of genital ulcers in different countries. Throughout South-East Asia and most parts of Africa, chancroid is the most common cause of genital ulcers, while syphilis and other infections are also relatively frequent (9–14). A small clinical study was conducted in Swaziland, using optimal laboratory support, to identify the etiology of ulcers (7). Chancroid accounted for 42% of the diagnoses, syphilis 16%, lymphogranuloma venereum 12%, and herpes simplex virus infection 11%. No bacteriological diagnosis could be established in 15% of genital ulcers. The investigators felt that the majority of this group are probably also chancroid or mixed infections, since the culture method used for *H. ducreyi* recovery was not optimal.

## 3. Patient care strategy

Genital ulcers can be categorized clinically as vesicular lesions and superficial erosions (herpes), single, painless ulcers without suppurative

---

[1] Adapted from Meheus (1)

## Fig. 5.  Genital ulcer protocol

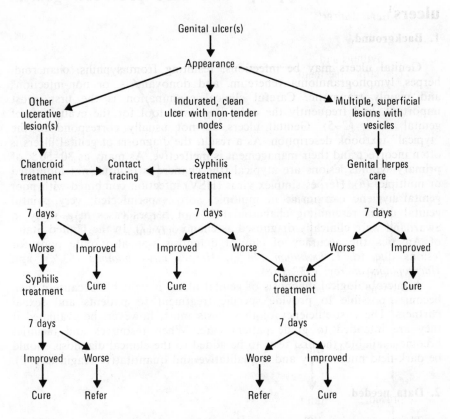

lymphadenopathy (syphilis), and other ulcerative lesions (Fig. 5). Without laboratory support, chancroid and syphilis are the two sexually transmitted diseases that can be treated; treatment should be as shown in the protocol.

## 4. Experience

This schedule is a slight modification of the one implemented in rural Swaziland in 1978. During this trial period, sulfadimidine was used to treat chancroid rather than cotrimoxazole. During one year 637 patients (464 males and 173 females) with genital ulcer(s) were seen representing 4 % of all consultations. This strategy was ineffective primarily because patient compliance with the sulfadimidine regimen of 4 doses daily for 7–10 days, was probably quite poor and *H. ducreyi* strains are rather insensitive to this drug (*15*).

Alternative approaches to the management of patients with genital ulcer disease can be proposed and evaluated. In African countries where both syphilis and chancroid are common, it has been suggested that a simpler

Fig. 6.   Simplified genital ulcer protocol

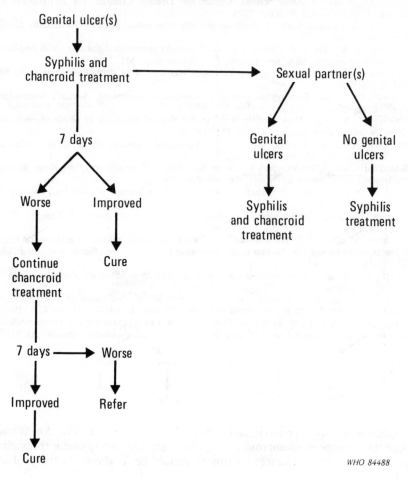

WHO 84488

protocol could be used (Fig. 6) (*16*). All patients with ulcers would receive combined treatment for chancroid and syphilis. Sexual partners with no ulcers would receive treatment for syphilis only, while partners with ulcers would receive combined treatment. This protocol has not yet been evaluated.

## References

1. MEHEUS, A. Z. Practical approaches in developing countries. In: Holmes, K. K. et al., ed. *Sexually transmitted diseases.* New York, McGraw-Hill, 1984.
2. WHO Technical Report Series, No. 660, 1981 (*Nongonococcal urethritis and other selected sexually transmitted diseases of public health importance:* report of a WHO scientific group).

3. HART, G. *Notes on penile lesions.* Center for Disease Control, US Department of Health, Education and Welfare, 1975.

4. STOLZ, E. & VAN DER STEK, J. *Portfolio sexually transmitted diseases.* Rotterdam, C. H. Boehringer Sohn, 1977.

5. MEHEUS, A. & URSI, J. P. *Clinical aspects of sexually transmitted diseases – with emphasis on genital ulceration:* Slide set. Upjohn Co., Kalamazoo, MI, 1981.

6. ANDERSON, K. E. The painful, non-indurated chancre. *Acta dermato-venereologica,* **58**: 554–555 (1978).

7. MEHEUS, A. ET AL. Etiology of genital ulcerations in Swaziland. *Sexually transmitted diseases,* **10**: 33–35 (1983).

8. CHAPEL, T. A. ET AL. How reliable is the morphological diagnosis of penile ulcerations? *Sexually transmitted diseases,* **4**: 150–152 (1977).

9. MEHEUS, A. ET AL. Genital infections in Swaziland. *Annales de la Société belge de médecine tropicale,* **62**: 361–367 (1982).

10. KIBUKAMUSOKE, J. W. Venereal disease in East Africa. *Transactions of the Royal Society of Tropical Medicine and Hygiene,* **59**: 642–648 (1965).

11. TAN, T. ET AL. Chancroid: a study of 500 cases. *Asian journal of infectious diseases,* **1**: 27–28 (1977).

12. NSANZE, H. ET AL. Genital ulcers in Kenya. *British journal of venereal diseases,* **57**: 378–381 (1981).

13. DUNCAN, M. O. ET AL. The diagnosis of sexually acquired genital ulcerations in black patients in Johannesburg. *Southern African journal of sexually transmitted diseases,* **1**: 20–23 (1981).

14. LATIF, A. S. Sexually transmitted disease in clinic patients in Salisbury, Zimbabwe. *British journal of venereal diseases,* **57**: 181–183 (1981).

15. FAST, M. ET AL. Antimicrobial therapy of chancroid: an evaluation of five treatment regimens correlated with *in vitro* sensitivity. *Sexually transmitted diseases,* **10**: 1–6 (1983).

16. AFRICAN UNION AGAINST VENEREAL DISEASES AND TREPONEMATOSES. *Recommendations for the therapy of genital ulcer disease in Africa.* Special document, Nairobi, AUVDT, 1983.

# Annex 5. Alternative uses of evaluation studies

1. *Using evaluation to attract attention to a problem.* Some examples of this approach are the cost-benefit analysis of syphilis control programmes done by Klarman (*1*), the exhortation by Callin about the costs of inadequate syphilis programmes (*2*), and the papers on the economic consequences of PID by Rendtorff et al. (*3*) and Curran (*4*).

2. *Pointing out the inefficiency or ineffectiveness of a case-finding procedure on certain population groups.* This point is illustrated by a report against routine screening for sexually transmitted disease of hospitalized elderly patients (*5*), studies signalling the lack of results of the 3-month follow-up serology on patients with gonorrhoea (*6*), the futility of taking rectal cultures in asymptomatic or heterosexual Danish males (*7*), and the ineffectiveness of rescreening for gonorrhoea in a Colorado clinic (*8*).

3. *"Effectiveness" is in the eyes of the beholder (or decision-maker).* A cost-effectiveness analysis of Swiss women cultured routinely for gonorrhoea was found cost-effective despite the low prevalence (0.81 %) of the disease (*9*), whereas, in the United States of America several studies (*10*, *11*) have advocated "selective" instead of routine screening in females with a low prevalence of gonorrhoea (between 1 and 4 %).

4. *Evaluation of changes in yield of gonorrhoea detection* by culturing other sites or by taking duplicate cultures is illustrated in reports by Keith et al. (*12*) and Dans & Judson (*13*).

5. *Evaluations of efficacy of treatment and of diagnostic tests* are covered in reports by Guinan et al. (*14*) and Rothenberg et al. (*15*).

6. *Training and patient management.* The use of protocols or algorithms in the management of disease is illustrated in the report by Rhodes et al. (*16*). Lee and Sparling's algorithms for syphilis could also serve this purpose (*17*).

7. *Extension of control activities.* The provocative editorial by Handsfield et al. (*18*) and the study by Willcox et al. (*19*) make the point that the time is right to use chlamydial cultures in countries which can afford them. The paper by Grady (*20*) regarding new approaches to hepatitis B prevention merits careful reading.

8. *The effectiveness of counselling* and other behavioural approaches for securing the patient's cooperation is illustrated by Kroger (*21*). The study by Potterat and Rothenberg (*22*) on contact-tracing should be repeated especially in developing countries where these activities are often négligible. A series of papers (*23–25*) evaluate the types of contacts which will benefit more by epidemiological investigation (males more than females) in certain settings.

9. *The studies on evaluation of venereal disease telephone answering services* (*26–28*) illustrate some of the difficulties in evaluating the impact of a new procedure.

10. *Using a decision-analytic approach,* Johnson (*29*) found justification for treating contacts on epidemiological grounds, and Rein (*30*) assessed strategies for the management of urethritis to decide which antibiotic regimen would be the most cost-effective.

11. Some papers raise questions regarding *policies which have become law*, such as the mandatory premarital syphilis serology (*31*).

Although this is not an exhaustive list and some of the analyses are incomplete or misdirected, these types of evaluations can be helpful in guiding policy and administrative decisions.

## References

1. KLARMAN, H. E. Syphilis control programs. In: Dorfman, H., ed. *Measuring the benefits of government investments.* Washington DC, The Brookings Institution, 1965.
2. CALLIN, A. E. Cuanto le cuesta a un país un programa inadecuado de control de sifilis? *Salud pública de México,* **10**: 611–614 (1968).
3. RENDTORFF, R. C. ET AL. Economic consequences of gonorrhoea in women: experience from an urban hospital. *Journal of the American Venereal Disease Association,* **1**: 40–47 (1974).
4. CURRAN, J. W. Economic consequences of pelvic inflammatory disease in the United States. *American journal of obstetrics and gynecology,* **138**: 848–851 (1980).
5. KIRKLAND, L. R. Syphilis surveillance (letter). *Journal of the American Medical Association,* **238**: 399 (1977).
6. WANSCHER, B. & KNUDSEN, L. Wassermann-Kontrol efter gonoré. *Ugeskrift for laeger,* **139**: 2987–2989 (1977).
7. WULF, H. C. Rektal gonoré. Nyttevirkningsanalyse af podning fra analkanalen. *Ugeskrift for laeger,* **141**: 3168–3170 (1979).
8. JUDSON, F. N. & WOLF, F. C. Rescreening for gonorrhoea: An evaluation of compliance methods and results. *American journal of public health,* **69**: 1178–1180 (1979).
9. LANDOLT, A. ET AL. Der kulturelle Gonokokken Nachweis: Eine Kosten–Nutzen–Analyse an einem geburtshilflich gynäkologischen Patientengut. *Geburtshilfe und Frauenheilkunde,* **38**: 255–259 (1978).
10. HINDS, M. W. Gonorrhoea screening in family planning clinics. When should it become selective? *Public health reports,* **92**: 361–364 (1977).
11. DUFF, P. An evaluation of routine screening for gonorrhoea in a population of military dependents. *Military medicine,* **144**: 322–325 (1979).
12. KEITH, L. ET AL. Gonorrhoea detection in a family planning clinic: A cost-benefit analysis of 2000 triplicate cultures. *American journal of obstetrics and gynecology,* **121**: 399–404 (1975).
13. DANS, P. E. & JUDSON, F. The establishment of a venereal disease clinic: II. An appraisal of current diagnostic methods in uncomplicated urogenital and rectal gonorrhoea. *Journal of American Venereal Disease Association,* **1**: 107–112 (1975).
14. GUINAN, M. E. ET AL. The national gonorrhoea therapy monitoring study: Review of treatment results and of in-vitro antibiotic susceptibility, 1972–1978. *Sexually transmitted diseases,* **6**: 93–102 (1979).
15. ROTHENBERG, R. B. ET AL. Efficacy of selected diagnostic tests for sexually transmitted diseases. *Journal of the American Medical Association,* **235**: 49–51 (1976).
16. RHODES, A. ET AL. Protocol management of male genitourinary infections. *Journal of American Venereal Disease Association,* **2**: 23–30 (1976).
17. LEE, T. J. & SPARLING, F. Syphilis. An algorithm. *Journal of the American Medical Association,* **242**: 1187–1189 (1979).
18. HANDSFIELD, H. H. ET AL. Public health implications and control of sexually transmitted chlamydial infections. *Sexually transmitted diseases,* **8**: 85–86 (1981).
19. WILLCOX, J. R. ET AL. The need for a chlamydial culture service. *British journal of venereal diseases,* **55**: 281–283 (1979).
20. GRADY, G. F. Strategies for prevention of hepatitis B as a sexually transmitted disease. *Sexually transmitted diseases,* **8**: 344–348 (1981).
21. KROGER, F. Compliance strategies in a clinic for treatment of sexually transmitted diseases. *Sexually transmitted diseases,* **7**: 178–182 (1980).

22. POTTERAT, J. J. & ROTHENBERG, R. The case-finding effectiveness of a self-referral system for gonorrhoea: A preliminary report. *American journal of public health*, **67**: 174–176 (1977).

23. BLOUNT, J. H. A new approach for gonorrhoea epidemiology. *American journal of public health*, **62**: 710–712 (1972).

24. BLOUNT, J. H. Gonorrhoea epidemiology: Insuring the best return for resources expended. *Journal of reproductive medicine*, **11**: 125–128 (1973).

25. MARINO, A. F. ET AL. Gonorrhoea epidemiology – is it worthwhile? *American journal of public health*, **62**: 713–714 (1972).

26. BRYANT, N. H. ET AL. VD Hotline: An evaluation. *Public health reports*, **91**: 231–235 (1976).

27. MORRISON, G. D. ET AL. A survey of the effectiveness of a telephone-answering service. *British journal of venereal diseases*, **54**: 344–345 (1978).

28. SCHUURMAN, J. H. ET AL. Effects of the automatic telephone answering service on venereal disease in Rotterdam. *Health education journal*, **39**: 47–51 (1980).

29. JOHNSON, R. E. Epidemiologic and prophylactic treatment of gonorrhoea: A decision analysis review. *Sexually transmitted diseases*, **6**: 159–167 (1979).

30. REIN, M. F. Therapeutic decisions in the treatment of sexually transmitted diseases: An overview. *Sexually transmitted diseases*, **8**: 93–99 (1981).

31. FELMAN, Y. M. Should premarital syphilis serologies continue to be mandated by law? *Journal of the American Medical Association*, **240**: 459–460 (1978).

# Annex 6. List of participants*

Michael Adler, Professor of Genitourinary Medicine, The Middlesex Hospital Medical School, James Pringle House, London, England (*Chairman*)

Juan Jose Apolinaire, Deputy Director of Hygiene and Epidemiology, Province of Cienfuegos, Cuba

F. John Bennett, Regional Adviser in Community Health, United Nations Children's Fund (UNICEF), Nairobi, Kenya

Claude Betts, Epidemiologist, Ministry of Health, Panama, Republic of Panama

Stuart T. Brown, Associate Director, Division of Venereal Disease Control, Centers for Disease Control, Atlanta, Georgia, USA (*Rapporteur*)

Georges Causse, Chief Medical Officer, Division of Communicable Diseases, World Health Organization, Geneva, Switzerland

William W. Darrow, Research Sociologist, Division of Venereal Disease Control, Centers for Disease Control, Atlanta, Georgia, USA

G. Elste, Physician-in-Chief, Dermatology Clinic, State Clinical Services, Berlin-Buch, German Democratic Republic

Gavin Hart, Senior Medical Specialist, Planning Department, South Australian Health Commission, Adelaide, South Australia, Australia (*Rapporteur*)

Orlando Jaramillo, Director, National Centre for Training and Research in Health and Social Security (CENDEISSS), San Jose, Costa Rica

Yamil Kouri, Director, Venereal Disease Control Program, San Juan, Puerto Rico, USA

Andre Meheus, Associate Professor of Epidemiology and Social Medicine, University of Antwerp, Wilrijk, Belgium (*Rapporteur*)

Charles Mertens, Professor of Medical Psychology, University of Louvain, Belgium, Visiting Professor in Behavioral Sciences, Harvard University, Boston, Massachusetts, USA

Herbert Nsanze, Chief, Department of Medical Microbiology, Faculty of Medicine, University of Nairobi, Nairobi, Kenya

A. Olu Osoba, Professor and Head, Department of Medical Microbiology, University College Hospital, Ibadan, Nigeria (*Vice-Chairman*)

David G. Ostrow, Medical Director, Howard Brown Memorial Clinic, Chicago, Illinois, USA

V. S. Rajan, Director, Middle Road Hospital, Singapore, Singapore (*Vice-Chairman*)

Richard Rothenberg, State Epidemiologist, Director, Bureau of Chronic Disease Prevention, New York State Department of Health, Albany, New York, USA

---

* Unable to attend: Sosroamijoyo Sudarto, Director for the Control of Diseases with Direct Transmission, CDC, Ministry of Health, Jakarta, Indonesia.

Ronald K. St John, Coordinator, Epidemiology Unit, Pan American Health Organization, Washington, DC, USA

E. H. Sng, Consultant Immunologist, Outram Road Hospital, Department of Pathology, Singapore, Singapore

Ken Sorungbe, Chief, Federal Epidemiological Unit, Federal Ministry of Health, Lagos, Nigeria

Keith Tones, Principal Lecturer, Health Education, Leeds Polytechnic, Leeds, England

Amnuay Traisupa, Director, Venereal Disease Division, Bangrak Hospital, Bangkok, Thailand

Paul J. Wiesner, Director, Chronic Diseases Division, Centers for Disease Control, Atlanta, Georgia, USA

Fernando Zacarias, Visiting Scientist, Division of Venereal Disease Control, Centers for Disease Control, Atlanta, Georgia, USA

Ronald K. St. John, Coordinator, Epidemiology Unit, Pan American Health Organization, Washington, DC, USA

E. H. Sng, Consultant Immunologist, Outram Road Hospital, Department of Pathology, Singapore

Ken Sorongbe, Chief, Federal Epidemiological Unit, Federal Ministry of Health, Lagos, Nigeria

Keith Tones, Principal Lecturer, Health Education, Leeds Polytechnic, Leeds, England

Annuay Trairatra, Director, Venereal Disease Division, Bangrak Hospital, Bangkok, Thailand

Paul J. Wiesner, Director, Chronic Diseases Division, Centers for Disease Control, Atlanta, Georgia, USA

Fernando Zacarias, Visiting Scientist, Division of Venereal Disease Control, Centers for Disease Control, Atlanta, Georgia, USA

WHO publications may be obtained, direct or through booksellers, from:

| | |
|---|---|
| ALGERIA | Société Nationale d'Edition et de Diffusion, 3 bd Zirout Youcef, ALGIERS |
| ARGENTINA | Carlos Hirsch SRL, Florida 165, Galerías Güemes, Escritorio 453/465, BUENOS AIRES |
| AUSTRALIA | Hunter Publications, 58A Gipps Street, COLLINGWOOD, VIC 3066 — Australian Government Publishing Service *(Mail order sales)*, P.O. Box 84, CANBERRA A.C.T. 2600; *or over the counter from:* Australian Government Publishing Service Bookshops *at:* 70 Alinga Street, CANBERRA CITY A.C.T. 2600; 294 Adelaide Street, BRISBANE, Queensland 4000; 347 Swanston Street, MELBOURNE, VIC 3000; 309 Pitt Street, SYDNEY, N.S.W. 2000; Mt Newman House, 200 St. George's Terrace, PERTH, WA 6000; Industry House, 12 Pirie Street, ADELAIDE, SA 5000; 156–162 Macquarie Street, HOBART, TAS 7000 — R. Hill & Son Ltd., 608 St. Kilda Road, MELBOURNE, VIC 3004; Lawson House, 10–12 Clark Street, CROW'S NEST, NSW 2065 |
| AUSTRIA | Gerold & Co., Graben 31, 1011 VIENNA I |
| BANGLADESH | The WHO Programme Coordinator, G.P.O. Box 250, DHAKA 5 — The Association of Voluntary Agencies, P.O. Box 5045, DHAKA 5 |
| BELGIUM | *For books:* Office International de Librairie s.a., avenue Marnix 30, 1050 BRUSSELS. *For periodicals and subscriptions:* Office International des Périodiques, avenue Marnix 30, 1050 BRUSSELS — *Subscriptions to World Health only:* Jean de Lannoy, 202 avenue du Roi, 1060 BRUSSELS |
| BHUTAN | *see* India, WHO Regional Office |
| BOTSWANA | Botsalo Books (Pty) Ltd., P.O. Box 1532, GABORONE |
| BRAZIL | Biblioteca Regional de Medicina OMS/OPS, Unidade de Venda de Publicações, Caixa Postal 20.381, Vila Clementino, 04023 SÃO PAULO, S.P. |
| BURMA | *see* India, WHO Regional Office |
| CANADA | Canadian Public Health Association, 1335 Carling Avenue, Suite 210, OTTAWA, Ont. K1Z 8N8. *Subscription orders, accompanied by cheque made out to the* Royal Bank of Canada, Ottawa, Account World Health Organization, *may also be sent to the* World Health Organization, PO Box 1800, Postal Station B, OTTAWA, Ont. K1P 5R5 |
| CHINA | China National Publications Import & Export Corporation, P.O. Box 88, BEIJING (PEKING) |
| CYPRUS | "MAM", P.O. Box 1722, NICOSIA |
| CZECHO-SLOVAKIA | Artia, Ve Smeckach 30, 111 27 PRAGUE 1 |
| DEMOCRATIC PEOPLE'S REPUBLIC OF KOREA | *see* India, WHO Regional Office |
| DENMARK | Munksgaard Export and Subscription Service, Nørre Søgade 35, 1370 COPENHAGEN K (Tel: +45 1 12 85 70) |
| ECUADOR | Libreria Científica S.A., P.O. Box 362, Luque 223, GUAYAQUIL |
| EGYPT | Osiris Office for Books and Reviews, 50 Kasr El Nil Street, CAIRO |
| FIJI | The WHO Programme Coordinator, P.O. Box 113, SUVA |
| FINLAND | Akateeminen Kirjakauppa, Keskuskatu 2, 00101 HELSINKI 10 |
| FRANCE | Librairie Arnette, 2 rue Casimir-Delavigne, 75006 PARIS |
| GABON | Librairie Universitaire du Gabon, B.P. 3881, LIBREVILLE |
| GERMAN DEMOCRATIC REPUBLIC | Buchhaus Leipzig, Postfach 140, 701 LEIPZIG |
| GERMANY, FEDERAL REPUBLIC OF | Govi-Verlag GmbH, Ginnheimerstrasse 20, Postfach 5360, 6236 ESCHBORN — W. E. Saarbach, Postfach 101 610, Follerstrasse 2, 5000 COLOGNE 1 — Alex. Horn, Spiegelgasse 9, Postfach 3340, 6200 WIESBADEN |
| GHANA | Fides Enterprises, P.O. Box 1628, ACCRA |
| GREECE | G.C. Eleftheroudakis S.A., Librairie internationale, rue Nikis 4, ATHENS (T. 126) |
| HAITI | Max Bouchereau, Librairie "A la Caravelle", Boîte postale 111-B, PORT-AU-PRINCE |
| HONG KONG | Hong Kong Government Information Services, Beaconsfield House, 6th Floor, Queen's Road, Central, VICTORIA |
| HUNGARY | Kultura, P.O.B. 149, BUDAPEST 62 — Akadémiai Könyvesbolt, Váci utca 22, BUDAPEST V |
| ICELAND | Snaebjørn Jonsson & Co., P.O. Box 1131, Hafnarstraeti 9, REYKJAVIK |
| INDIA | WHO Regional Office for South-East Asia, World Health House, Indraprastha Estate, Mahatma Gandhi Road, NEW DELHI 110002 — Oxford Book & Stationery Co., Scindia House, NEW DELHI 110001; 17 Park Street, CALCUTTA 700016 *(Sub-agent)* |
| INDONESIA | P. T. Kalman Media Pusaka, Pusat Perdagangan Senen, Block 1, 4th Floor, P.O. Box 3433/Jkt, JAKARTA |
| IRAN (ISLAMIC REPUBLIC OF) | Iran University Press, 85 Park Avenue, P.O. Box 54/551, TEHRAN |
| IRAQ | Ministry of Information, National House for Publishing, Distributing and Advertising, BAGHDAD |
| IRELAND | TDC Publishers, 12 North Frederick Street, DUBLIN 1 (Tel: 744835–749677) |
| ISRAEL | Heiliger & Co., 3 Nathan Strauss Street, JERUSALEM 94227 |
| ITALY | Edizioni Minerva Medica, Corso Bramante 83–85, 10126 TURIN; Via Lamarmora 3, 20100 MILAN |
| JAPAN | Maruzen Co. Ltd., P.O. Box 5050, TOKYO International, 100–31 |
| JORDAN, THE HASHEMITE KINGDOM OF | Jordan Book Centre Co. Ltd., University Street, P.O. Box 301 (Al-Jubeiha), AMMAN |
| KUWAIT | The Kuwait Bookshops Co. Ltd., Thunayan Al-Ghanem Bldg, P.O. Box 2942, KUWAIT |
| LAO PEOPLE'S DEMOCRATIC REPUBLIC | The WHO Programme Coordinator, P.O. Box 343, VIENTIANE |
| LEBANON | The Levant Distributors Co. S.A.R.L., Box 1181, Makdassi Street, Hanna Bldg, BEIRUT |
| LUXEMBOURG | Librairie du Centre, 49 bd Royal, LUXEMBOURG |
| MALAWI | Malawi Book Service, P.O. Box 30044, Chichiti, BLANTYRE 3 |

WHO publications may be obtained, direct or through booksellers, from:

| | |
|---|---|
| MALAYSIA | The WHO Programme Coordinator, Room 1004, 10th Floor, Wisma Lim Foo Yong (formerly Fitzpatrick's Building), Jalan Raja Chulan, KUALA LUMPUR 05–10; P.O. Box 2550, KUALA LUMPUR 01–02; Parry's Book Center, K. L. Hilton Hotel, Jln. Treacher, P.O. Box 960, KUALA LUMPUR |
| MALDIVES | *see* India, WHO Regional Office |
| MEXICO | Libreria Internacional, S.A. de C.V., Av. Sonora 206, 06100-MÉXICO, D.F. |
| MONGOLIA | *see* India, WHO Regional Office |
| MOROCCO | Editions La Porte, 281 avenue Mohammed V, RABAT |
| MOZAMBIQUE | INLD, Caixa Postal 4030, MAPUTO |
| NEPAL | *see* India, WHO Regional Office |
| NETHERLANDS | Medical Books Europe BV, Noorderwal 38, 7241 BL LOCHEM |
| NEW ZEALAND | Government Printing Office, Publications Section, Mulgrave Street, Private Bag, WELLINGTON 1; Walter Street, WELLINGTON; World Trade Building, Cubacade, Cuba Street, WELLINGTON. *Government Bookshops at:* Hannaford Burton Building, Rutland Street, Private Bag, AUCKLAND; 159 Hereford Street, Private Bag, CHRISTCHURCH; Alexandra Street, P.O. Box 857, HAMILTON; T & G Building, Princes Street, P.O. Box 1104, DUNEDIN — R. Hill & Son Ltd, Ideal House, Cnr Gillies Avenue & Eden Street, Newmarket, AUCKLAND 1 |
| NIGERIA | University Bookshop Nigeria Ltd, University of Ibadan, IBADAN |
| NORWAY | J. G. Tanum A/S, P.O. Box 1177 Sentrum, OSLO 1 |
| PAKISTAN | Mirza Book Agency, 65 Shahrah-E-Quaid-E-Azam, P.O. Box 729, LAHORE 3; Sasi Limited, Sasi Centre, G.P.O. Box 779, I.I. Chundrigar Road, KARACHI |
| PAPUA NEW GUINEA | The WHO Programme Coordinator, P.O. Box 646, KONEDOBU |
| PHILIPPINES | World Health Organization, Regional Office for the Western Pacific, P.O. Box 2932, MANILA — The Modern Book Company Inc., P.O. Box 632, 922 Rizal Avenue, MANILA 2800 |
| POLAND | Składnica Księgarska, ul Mazowiecka 9, 00052 WARSAW *(except periodicals)* — BKWZ Ruch, ul Wronia 23, 00840 WARSAW *(periodicals only)* |
| PORTUGAL | Livraria Rodrigues, 186 Rua do Ouro, LISBON 2 |
| REPUBLIC OF KOREA | The WHO Programme Coordinator, Central P.O. Box 540, SEOUL |
| SIERRA LEONE | Njala University College Bookshop (University of Sierra Leone), Private Mail Bag, FREETOWN |
| SINGAPORE | The WHO Programme Coordinator, 144 Moulmein Road, SINGAPORE 1130; Newton P.O. Box 31, SINGAPORE 9122 — Select Books (Pte) Ltd, 215 Tanglin Shopping Centre, 2/F, 19 Tanglin Road, SINGAPORE 10 |
| SOUTH AFRICA | Van Schaik's Bookstore (Pty) Ltd, P.O. Box 724, 268 Church Street, PRETORIA 0001 |
| SPAIN | Comercial Atheneum S.A., Consejo de Ciento 130–136, BARCELONA 15; General Moscardó 29, MADRID 20 — Librería Diaz de Santos, Lagasca 95 y Maldonado 6, MADRID 6; Balmes 417 y 419, BARCELONA 22 |
| SRI LANKA | *see* India, WHO Regional Office |
| SWEDEN | *For books:* Aktiebolaget C.E. Fritzes Kungl. Hovbokhandel, Regeringsgatan 12, 103 27 STOCKHOLM. *For periodicals:* Wennergren-Williams AB, Box 30004, 104 25 STOCKHOLM |
| SWITZERLAND | Medizinischer Verlag Hans Huber, Länggass Strasse 76, 3012 BERNE 9 |
| THAILAND | *see* India, WHO Regional Office |
| TUNISIA | Société Tunisienne de Diffusion, 5 avenue de Carthage, TUNIS |
| TURKEY | Haset Kitapevi, 469 Istiklal Caddesi, Beyoglu, ISTANBUL |
| UNITED KINGDOM | H.M. Stationery Office: 49 High Holborn, LONDON WC1V 6HB; 13a Castle Street, EDINBURGH EH2 3AR; 80 Chichester Street, BELFAST BT1 4JY; Brazennose Street, MANCHESTER M60 8AS; 258 Broad Street, BIRMINGHAM B1 2HE; Southey House, Wine Street, BRISTOL BS1 2BQ. *All mail orders should be sent to:* HMSO Publications Centre, 51 Nine Elms Lane, LONDON SW8 5DR |
| UNITED STATES OF AMERICA | *Single and bulk copies of individual publications (not subscriptions):* WHO Publications Centre USA, 49 Sheridan Avenue, ALBANY, NY 12210. *Subscriptions: Subscription orders, accompanied by check made out to the* Chemical Bank, New York, Account World Health Organization, *should be sent to the* World Health Organization, PO Box 5284, Church Street Station, NEW YORK, NY 10249; *Correspondence concerning subscriptions should be addressed to the* World Health Organization, Distribution and Sales, 1211 GENEVA 27, Switzerland. *Publications are also available from the* United Nations Bookshop, NEW YORK, NY 10017 *(retail only)* |
| URUGUAY | Libreria Agropecuaria S. R. L., Casilla de Correo 1755, Alzaibar 1328, MONTEVIDEO |
| USSR | *For readers in the USSR requiring Russian editions:* Komsomolskij prospekt 18, Medicinskaja Kniga, Moscow — *For readers outside the USSR requiring Russian editions:* Kuzneckij most 18, Meždunarodnaja Kniga, Moscow G-200 |
| VENEZUELA | Libreria del Este, Apartado 60.337, CARACAS 106 — Libreria Médica Paris, Apartado 60.681, CARACAS 106 |
| YUGOSLAVIA | Jugoslovenska Knjiga, Terazije 27/II, 11000 BELGRADE |
| ZAIRE | Librairie universitaire, avenue de la Paix No 167, B.P. 1682, KINSHASA I |

Special terms for developing countries are obtainable on application to the WHO Programme Coordinators or WHO Regional Offices listed above or to the World Health Organization, Distribution and Sales Service, 1211 Geneva 27, Switzerland. Orders from countries where sales agents have not yet been appointed may also be sent to the Geneva address, but must be paid for in pounds sterling, US dollars, or Swiss francs.

Price: Sw. fr. 14.—                    Prices are subject to change without notice.

300101150B